Mortality of Veteran Participants in the CROSSROADS Nuclear Test

Medical Follow-up Agency

INSTITUTE OF MEDICINE

by
J. Christopher Johnson
Susan Thaul
William F. Page
Harriet Crawford

with oversight from the

Institute of Medicine
Committee on the CROSSROADS Nuclear Test

NATIONAL ACADEMY PRESS
Washington, D.C. 1996

National Academy Press • 2101 Constitution Avenue, N.W. • Washington, DC 20418

NOTICE: The project that is the subject of this report was approved by the Governing Board of the National Research Council, whose members are drawn from the councils of the National Academy of Sciences, the National Academy of Engineering, and the Institute of Medicine. The members of the committee responsible for the report were chosen for their special competencies and with regard for appropriate balance.

This report has been reviewed by a group other than the authors according to procedures approved by a Report Review Committee consisting of members of the National Academy of Sciences, the National Academy of Engineering, and the Institute of Medicine.

The Institute of Medicine was chartered in 1970 by the National Academy of Sciences to enlist distinguished members of the appropriate professions in the examination of policy matters pertaining to the health of the public. In this, the Institute acts under both the Academy's 1863 congressional charter responsibility to be an adviser to the federal government and its own initiative in identifying issues of medical care, research, and education. Dr. Kenneth I. Shine is president of the Institute of Medicine.

Support for this project was provided by the U.S. Department of Veterans Affairs contract nos.V101(93)P1431 and V101(93)P1165), cofunded by the Defense Special Weapons Agency (formerly, Defense Nuclear Agency). This support does not constitute an endorsement of the views expressed in this report.

Library of Congress Catalog Card No. 96-71162
International Standard Book No. 0-309-05596-2
Additional copies of this report are available from:

National Academy Press
2101 Constitution Avenue, N.W.
Box 285
Washington, DC 20055

Call (800) 624-6242 or (202) 334-3313 (in the Washington metropolitan area), or visit the NAP's online bookstore at **http://www.nap.edu.**

Printed in the United States of America

The serpent has been a symbol of long life, healing, and knowledge among almost all cultures and religions since the beginning of recorded history. The serpent adopted as a logotype by the Institute of Medicine is a relief carving from ancient Greece, now held by the Staatlichemuseen in Berlin.

COMMITTEE ON THE CROSSROADS NUCLEAR TEST

RICHARD B. SETLOW, *Chair,* Associate Director for Life Sciences and Senior Biophysicist, Biology Department, Brookhaven National Laboratory, Upton, New York
GILBERT W. BEEBE, Statistician, Radiation Epidemiology Branch, National Cancer Institute, Bethesda, Maryland
RICHARD L. BOYLAN, Senior Military Reference Archivist, National Archives and Records Administration, College Park, Maryland
DANIEL H. FREEMAN, JR., Professor, Office of Biostatistics, University of Texas Medical Branch, Galveston, Texas
ETHEL S. GILBERT, Senior Staff Scientist and Statistician, Pacific Northwest Division, Battelle Memorial Institute, Richland, Washington
DENNIS F. HOEFFLER, Medical Director, General Electric Lighting, Cleveland, Ohio
BARBARA S. HULKA, Professor, Department of Epidemiology, University of North Carolina, Chapel Hill, North Carolina
KEITH J. SCHIAGER, Director Emeritus, Radiological Health Department, University of Utah, Salt Lake City, Utah
SEYMOUR JABLON, Radiation Epidemiology Branch, National Cancer Institute, Bethesda, Maryland (through 1/93)

Study Staff

J. CHRISTOPHER JOHNSON, Study Director
HARRIET CRAWFORD, Operations Team Leader
WILLIAM F. PAGE, Biostatistician
PAMELA C. RAMEY-McCRAY, Project Assistant
SUSAN THAUL, Epidemiologist
DENNIS ROBINETTE (through 12/91)
YOUN SHIM (6/94–1/95)

Preface

In November of 1983 the Congress of the United States passed Public Law 98-160 that directed the Veterans Administration (VA) to provide for the conduct of epidemiological studies of the long-term adverse health effects of exposure to ionizing radiation from detonation of nuclear devices. In response, the Medical Follow-up Agency (MFUA), then in the Commission on Life Sciences, National Academy of Sciences (NAS), proposed to compare the mortality experience of veteran participants in the CROSSROADS nuclear test to a similar group of nonparticipants. Operation CROSSROADS involved approximately 40,000 military personnel, mostly Navy, and occurred in July of 1946 at the Bikini Atoll in the Marshall Islands.

The VA convened an *ad hoc* scientific committee to review the NAS proposal which they recommended should be funded to "enlarge the growing body of information relating to the effects of low levels of radiation on human populations." The study was begun in September of 1986 and in 1988, a committee of the Institute of Medicine was organized to provide guidance and advice to the MFUA staff on the conduct of the study. The study was interrupted by the untimely death of the principal investigator, Dr. Dennis Robinette, in 1992. Both the Committee and MFUA staff wish to acknowledge their debt of gratitude to Dr. Robinette who laid the ground work for this study and assembled the comparison cohort. We regret he was not able to see the fruits of his labors in the publication of this report.

The Committee to Study the Crossroads Nuclear Test has met periodically since 1988 to review and guide the work of the MFUA staff as they have conducted the study. As with all research, resources are not boundless, and decisions must be made to apply them where the potential for gain is the greatest. This study is no exception. While servicemen from all services participated in Operation CROSSROADS about 91 percent were from the Navy and the rest were distributed among the Marine Corps and the Army, which then included the Air Force. We chose to concentrate on the Navy cohort, and the reader will find that the conclusions are based on that group alone. Detailed investigation of the remaining branches of service are left to other ongoing and future studies in which the populations of Army, Air Force and Marines are much larger.

Since this is a congressionally mandated study, we expect that these results will be of interest to a wide range of readers from epidemiologists and scientists, to policy makers, veterans, and interested but possibly nontechnical readers. To make the report useful to such a wide audience has been a challenge. Hopefully, the scientists will find the detail and rigor they are accustomed to seeing in a technical report, while the interested readers with training outside the sciences will find sufficient background material to enable them to follow the technical discussion and understand the findings in the context of standard epidemiologic methods.

Richard B. Setlow, *Chair*

Acknowledgments

The Committee and the authors wish to express their appreciation to the veterans, too numerous to thank individually, who have provided us with information on their participation in CROSSROADS and to the veterans' groups that represent them. We are particularly indebted to Mr. Boley Caldwell of the National Association of Atomic Veterans (NAAV), who gave us the list of CROSSROADS veterans that we used as one source in verifying our participant list; Dr. Oscar Rosen for his perspective on Operation CROSSROADS as a participant and Director of NAAV; Mr. Robert Campbell, for the relevant information and documents he has provided over the course of the study; and Mrs. Pat Broudy, for her insights on the legislative aspects of atomic veteran compensation programs.

We have performed this study under Department of Veterans Affairs (VA) contracts (V101(93)P1431 and V101(93)P1165) which were cofunded by the Defense Special Weapons Agency (DSWA). We are appreciative of their support. The DSWA also provided indispensable information about the participants in Operation CROSSROADS study from their Nuclear Test Personnel Review (NTPR) database. In addition to funding, the VA has provided support in ascertaining the mortality of the cohort.

We are also in the debt of the National Archives and particularly the National Personnel Records Center, St. Louis MO, and their staffs, who provided us with necessary individual, mortality and unit data. Dr. Eric Gunderson and Dr. Frank Garland of the Naval Health Research Center, San Diego, gave us much useful information on the classification of both ships and personnel within the Navy.

We particularly acknowledge the contributions of the Operations Team of the MFUA, for their untiring, behind-the-scenes work to compile, edit, endlessly query and maintain the files of nearly 80,000 veterans whose records make up the database for this study. Without their expertise and experience in building military study cohorts of this type, the CROSSROADS investigation would not have been possible. Finally, we thank Dr. Richard Miller, director MFUA for his assistance and encouragement, Mrs. Pamela Ramey-McCray for her administrative support, Ms. Nancy Diener for budgetary guidance, and Mr. Peter Slavin for his editorial review.

Glossary and Acronyms

ABLE. Military code name of 1 July 1946 nuclear detonation in Operation CROSSROADS.

AMFIT. A statistical modeling program (in the Epicure software package) used to compute standardized mortality ratios (SMRs) .

background radiation. Detected disintegration events not emanating from the sample. Natural background is that radiation that is a natural part of a person's environment, primarily terrestrial radioactivity and cosmic rays.

BAKER. Military code name of 25 July 1946 nuclear detonation in Operation CROSSROADS.

BEIR. Biological Effects of Ionizing Radiation: A series of reports by committees of the National Academy of Sciences.

BEIR IV. Biological Effects of Ionizing Radiation, 1988 Report IV (see References).

BEIR V. Biological Effects of Ionizing Radiation, 1990 Report V (see References).

BIRLS. Beneficiary Identification and Records Locator Subsystem, Department of Veterans Affairs.

BRER. Board on Radiation Effects Research, National Research Council.

CDC. Centers for Disease Control and Prevention, DHHS.

CFR. Code of Federal Regulations.

CI. Confidence interval (epidemiology/statistics).

CJTF-1. Commander, Joint Task Force One.

CLL. Chronic lymphocytic leukemia, a form of leukemia that has not been found in studies to be radiogenic.

CNS. Central nervous system.

cohort study. An epidemiologic investigation or follow-up of a group of individuals who are known to have had an exposure or a disease and whose health status is followed over time. Can usually provide a basis for calculating risk or disease outcome.

confounder. A variable that is causally related to the disease under study and is associated with exposure in the study population, but is not a consequence of this exposure.

CROSSROADS. Military code name of atmospheric test of nuclear weapons, July 1946, Bikini Atoll, Marshall Islands.

DD-214. Military service discharge form.

DHHS. Department of Health and Human Services, USA.

DNA. Defense Nuclear Agency. The name was changed to Defense Special Weapons Agency (DSWA) in June 1996.

DoD. Department of Defense, USA.

dose. The amount of absorbed radiation energy.

DSWA. Defense Special Weapons Agency (new name for DNA as of June 1996).

E1–E7. Enlisted personnel paygrades.

exposure (radiation). A term describing the amount of ionizing radiation that is incident upon living or inanimate material.

FARC. Federal Archives Records Center.

film badge. Photographic film shielded from light; worn by an individual to measure radiation exposure.

gamma ray. Radiation emitted from the nucleus having a wavelength range of 10^{-9}–10^{-12} centimeters.

GAO. General Accounting Office, USA.

HCFA. Health Care Financing Administration, DHHS.

ICD9. International Classification of Diseases, 9th revision. (See References, World Health Organization, 1995)

ICRP. International Commission on Radiological Protection.

incidence. The number of persons who have developed a disease in a given period of time divided by the total population at risk.

IOM. Institute of Medicine.

ionizing radiation. Radiation that produces ion pairs along its path through a substance.
irradiation. Exposure to radiation.

JTF. Joint task force.

LTFU. Lost to follow-up.

MFUA. Medical Follow-up Agency, Institute of Medicine.
mrem. Millirem, one-thousandth of a rem.
MSN. Military service number.
mSv. Millisievert, one-thousandth of a Sv.

NAAV. National Association of Atomic Veterans.
NARA. National Archives and Records Administration.
NAS. National Academy of Sciences.
NCRP. National Council on Radiation Protection and Measurements.
NDI. National Death Index, maintained by the National Center for Health Statistics, CDC, DHHS.
NPRC. National Personnel Records Center.
NRC. National Research Council.
NRC. Nuclear Regulatory Commission. United States government agency regulating by-product material.
NRPB. National Radiological Protection Board, U.K.
NTPR. Nuclear Test Personnel Review, DNA.

O1–O10. Commissioned officer paygrades.
odds ratio (OR). Used as an estimation of relative risk. Primarily used for case-control studies and is calculated from the odds of exposure among the cases to that among controls.
OTA. Office of Technology Assessment, U.S. Congress.

p. Probability (epidemiology/statistics, e.g., $p = .05$).
PHREG. Proportional hazards regression program, SAS.

radiation. Energy propagated through space or matter as waves (gamma rays, ultraviolet light) or as particles (alpha or beta rays). External radiation is from a source outside the body, whereas internal radiation is from a source inside the body (e.g., radionuclides deposited in tissues).
RADSAFE. Radiation safety monitor units, or personnel.
relative risk—RR. The ratio of the incidence of a condition in the exposed population divided by the incidence in the nonexposed population. If there is no difference as a result of exposure, the RR is 1.0.

rem. A unit of radiation dose equivalent; replaced by the sievert.
Roentgen (R). Quantity of x- or gamma radiation that produces one electrostatic unit of charge per cubic centimeter of air; a unit of exposure.

SAS. Originally "Statistical Analysis System," proprietary software package.
shield (shielding). A body of material used to reduce the intensity of radiation.
SI. International System of Units (as instituted in 1960).
sievert (Sv). A unit of effective or equivalent dose. Equivalent dose incorporates an adjustment for the fact that different types of radiation (alpha, beta, gamma, neutron) differ in their ability to do biologic damage. Effective dose also incorporates adjustments for the relative sensitivity of different organ systems. The sievert is the SI unit that replaced the rem.
SMR. Standardized mortality ratio.
SSN. Social Security Number.
Sv. sievert.

UNSCEAR. United Nations Scientific Committee on the Effects of Atomic Radiation. A committee of the U.N. General Assembly.
US. United States.
USS. United States Ship, Navy.

VA. Department of Veterans Affairs.
VAMI. Veterans Affairs (was Veterans Administration) Master Index.
VARO. Veterans Affairs Regional Office.

W1–W4. Warrant officer paygrades.

Contents

SUMMARY 1

1 STUDY RATIONALE AND OVERVIEW 4
Rationale, 4
Overview, 6

2 OTHER STUDIES OF THE HUMAN HEALTH EFFECTS OF RADIATION EXPOSURE 8

3 EPIDEMIOLOGY PRIMER 11
Choice of Comparison Group, 12
Fine Tuning of Exposed Group, 14
Confounders, 14
Data Collection, 15
Interpreting Data Findings, 17
Epidemiology Summary Related to this Study, 19

4 DESCRIPTION OF OPERATION CROSSROADS 21

5 DATA SOURCES FOR THE CROSSROADS STUDY 24

6 THE PARTICIPANT COHORT 27
Independent Verification of Participant Cohort, 29

Exclusion of "Post-Crossroads" Participants, 29
Crossroads Participants Who Participated in Other Nuclear Tests, 29
Primary Analysis—Navy Personnel Only, 30
Exclusivity of Participant and Comparison Cohorts, 30

7 THE COMPARISON COHORT 31
Comparison Cohort Selection, 31
Navy and Shipboard Marines, 31
Army and Army Air Corps, 33
Military Personnel Records, 33
Additional Controls, 34

8 EXPOSURE DEFINITION, MEASUREMENT, AND VERIFICATION 35
Introduction, 35
Dosimetry Background, 36
Definition of Potential Surrogate Dose Groups, 36
DNA-Provided Dose Estimates, 37
Participant versus Nonparticipant Cohorts as an Exposure Surrogate, 38
Boarders versus Nonboarding Participants versus Nonparticipants as Exposure Surrogates, 39
Engineering & Hull versus Other Specialty Status as an Exposure Surrogate, 39
Relationships of Surrogates with DNA Dose Data, 42
Decisions for the Analyses in this Report, 43

9 MORTALITY ASCERTAINMENT 44
Procedure, 45
Vital Status Ascertainment, 45
Cause and Date-of-Death Ascertainment, 46
Summary of Mortality Ascertainment Quality and Its Potential Effects on Valid Interpretation of the Findings, 46

10 CHARACTERIZATION OF THE COHORTS AND ANALYSIS PLAN 49
Data Decisions Taken Before Analysis, 49
Restricting Data Elements or Sample Definition, 49
Data Cleaning and Variable Development, 50
Univariate Descriptions of Study Population, 51
Missing Data, 53
Imputation of Fact and Date of Death, 53
Imputation of Date of Birth, 54
Summary, 54

Mortality Comparisons, 55
Multivariate Analyses, 56
Cox Proportional Hazards Model, 56
Standardized Mortality Ratios, 59
Analysis of Army (including Army Air Corps) and Marine Data, 60
Not the Subject of Analysis in this Report, 60

11 FINDINGS AND DISCUSSION 62
Organization, 62
Findings: Displayed in Tables, 64
Narrative Summary of Findings, 72
Participant Status, 72
Boarder Status/Hypothesized Exposure Gradient, 73
Engineering & Hull Status/Hypothesized Exposure Surrogate, 74
Findings for Marines and Army (including Army Air Corps) Personnel, 74
Discussion, 76
Boarders, 76
Engineering & Hull, 77
Discussion of Other Findings, 78
Other Models and Parameters Considered During Analysis, 79
Standardized Mortality Ratios, 81
Discussion Relating These Findings to Those of Similar Studies, 81
Findings in Other Studies of Atomic Veterans, 81
Selection Bias as an Explanation for Increased Participant All-Cause Mortality, 82
Avenues of Further Exploration, 84

12 CONCLUSIONS 86
Summary of Findings, 86

REFERENCES 89

APPENDIXES
A National Association of Atomic Veterans (NAAV) Medical Survey, 93
B Participant Description (DNA memorandum dated July 11, 1994), 99
C Standardized Mortality Ratios, 105
D Radiation Doses for CROSSROADS Participants and Exposure Surrogate Groups, 110
E Verification of Completeness and Accuracy of the Participant Roster, 114
F Verification of Completeness and Accuracy of Mortality Ascertainment, 128

List of Tables

TABLE 6-1. Distribution of Participation in Nuclear Test Series, 30

TABLE 8-1. Broad Occupational Specialty Groupings of Navy Enlisted Ratings Developed from "Navy Career Paths" (1949), 40
TABLE 8-2. General Rank/Rating and Occupational Specialty Categories for Navy Personnel, 41

TABLE 10-1. Age-at-Shot Distribution of Navy Participants and Controls, 51
TABLE 10-2. Distribution of Ranks and Ratings Among Navy Participants and Controls, 52
TABLE 10-3. Distribution of Occupational Specialties Among Navy Participants and Controls, 53
TABLE 10-4. Distribution of Boarders in the Study Cohort, 53
TABLE 10-5. Number and Percent of Records with Missing Needed Data Item, 54
TABLE 10-6. Vital Status on Follow-Up, 55
TABLE 10-7. Information Available on Deaths, 55
TABLE 10-8. Definitions of Analysis Variables, 57
TABLE 10-9. ICD9 Mortality Codes Used as Case Definitions for Analyses, 58

TABLE 11-1. Rate Ratios of Major Mortality Endpoints for Exposed to Not Exposed Personnel, 65
TABLE 11-2. Mortality Rate Ratios from Six Selected Major Cause-of-Death Categories (subset of Table 11-1), 66

TABLE 11-3. Mortality Rate Ratios from Remaining Major Cause-of-Death Categories (subset of Table 11-1), 67
TABLE 11-4. Mortality Rate Ratios from Selected Cancer Sites within All Malignancies (Table 11-2), 68
TABLE 11-5. Mortality Rate Ratios for Selected Cancer Sites within Digestive, Respiratory, and Lymphopoietic Cancers (subset of Table 11-4), 69
TABLE 11-6. Mortality Rate Ratio for Selected Subset of Other Lymphatic Tissue (subset of Table 11-5), 69
TABLE 11-7. Mortality Rate Ratios for Subset of External Causes (subset of Table 11-2), 70
TABLE 11-8. Mortality Rate Ratio for Subset of All Accidents (subset of Table 11-7), 71
TABLE 11-9. Rate Ratios for All-Cause Mortality of Engineering & Hull to Non-Engineering & Hull Groups by Status as Participants or Controls, 71
TABLE 11-10. Mortality Rate Ratios of Participants Relative to Controls (Marines, n = 1,137), 75
TABLE 11-11. Mortality Rate Ratios of Participants Relative to Controls (Army, including Army Air Corps, n = 6,482), 75
TABLE 11-12. Nonsignificant Risk Estimates from Tables 11-4 and 11-5 that Indicate at Least a 40 Percent Excess or Deficit in Mortality, 80
TABLE 11-13. All-Cause Mortality Rate Ratios, Including and Excluding Records with Imputed Dates of Birth, 80

TABLE C-1. Standardized Mortality Ratios for All Causes of Death in Navy Participants and Controls, 107
TABLE C-2. Standardized Mortality Ratios for All-Malignancy Deaths in Navy Participants and Controls, 108
TABLE C-3. Standardized Mortality Ratios (SMR) for Leukemia (including CLL) for Navy Enlisted Personnel (n = 66,831), 109
TABLE C-4. Standardized Mortality Ratios (SMR) for Army (including Army Air Corps, n = 6,482), 109
TABLE C-5. Standardized Mortality Ratios (SMR) for Marines (n = 1,137), 109

TABLE D-1. Tabulation of DNA Assigned Total Doses (rem [cSv]) by Study Grouping and Status as a Boarder or Nonboarder, 113

TABLE E-1. Resolution of 617 Apparent Participant Deletions Between 1986 and 1994, 119
TABLE E-2. Summary of Completeness of the NTPR Participant List as Indicated by Veteran Responses to MFUA Solicitations Published in Veterans' Publications, 121
TABLE E-3. Disposition of 103 Records of Putative Participants in CROSS-ROADS Whose Status Was Uncertain, 122

TABLE E-4. Disposition of 89 Discrepant Records from the NAAV Medical Survey List, 123
TABLE E-5. Summary of Completeness of the NTPR Participant List According to *Write-in* Data (includes verification of 17 discrepancies by personnel record searches at DNA), 123

TABLE F-1. Procedural Steps and Success Rates for Determination of Vital Status Information, 129
TABLE F-2. Vital Status for Navy Personnel, 130
TABLE F-3. Completeness of Mortality Information, 130
TABLE F-4. Summary of Vital Status for Study Records Submitted to HCFA, 131
TABLE F-5. Comparison of VA and HCFA Vital Status for Operation CROSSROADS Participants and Controls, 133
TABLE F-6. Number of Potential Matches for Each Record Submitted to NDI, 135
TABLE F-7. Comparison of NDI and MFUA Mortality Information, 136
TABLE F-8. NDI and HCFA Comparisons, 137
TABLE F-9. Distribution of Causes of Death for 641 Death Certificates Sent for Recoding, 138

Summary

Mortality experience was evaluated for the approximately 40,000 U.S. Navy personnel who participated in Operation CROSSROADS, a 1946 atmospheric nuclear test series that took place in the Bikini Atoll in the Marshall Islands. To judge whether that mortality experience was influenced by CROSSROADS participation, those personnel were compared to a control group assembled to be similar to the participants in all ways (age, paygrade, military service, time of service, location of service) possible except for Operation CROSSROADS participation.

A roster of CROSSROADS participants was assembled and provided to the Medical Follow-up Agency (MFUA) by the Nuclear Test Personnel Review (NTPR) program of the Defense Nuclear Agency.[1] A validation study by MFUA examining other sources of information regarding participant status found that the final roster captured between 93 and 99 percent of the military personnel who participated in Operation CROSSROADS. The mortality data gathered from Department of Veterans Affairs (VA) records were validated by sample comparisons with other national data sources. By the study cut-off date, 31 December 1992, 31.3 percent of the participants and 30.8 percent of the comparison cohort were known to have died. Cause of death was available for 86.3 percent of the participants and 89.3 percent of the controls.

Adjusting for remaining differences between the cohorts in distributions of age and paygrade, we compared, using proportional hazards analysis, the survival times of the two groups. Because available dosimetry data were not considered suitable for epidemiologic analysis, we based this study on exposure

[1]In June 1996 the Defense Nuclear Agency became the Defense Special Weapons Agency.

surrogate groups. We looked at three principal causes of mortality: all-cause, all-cancer, and leukemia, hypothesizing that increases in the latter two could result from radiation exposure. For descriptive purposes we also present comparisons between participants and the comparison group for 44 other disease categories. Findings stated in this report follow.

• Among Navy personnel, the primary analysis group for this study, we found that participants at the CROSSROADS nuclear test experienced higher mortality than a comparable group of nonparticipating military controls. The increase in all-cause mortality was 4.6 percent (relative risk [RR] = 1.046, 95% confidence interval, 1.020–1.074) and was statistically significant ($p < 0.001$).[2] For malignancies, the elevation of mortality was lower—RR = 1.014 (0.96–1.068)—and was not statistically significant ($p = 0.26$). Similarly, leukemia mortality RR was elevated to 1.020 (0.75–1.39), but not significantly ($p = 0.90$) and by less than all-cause mortality. The increase in all-cause mortality did not appear to concentrate in any of the disease groups we considered. Of the 44 other specific cancers and disease categories we examined, there were no statistically significant increases in mortality. The overall elevation of mortality rate ratios for malignancies and leukemias in the participants were not statistically significant and, in fact, were lower than for many other causes of death.

• Navy mortality due to all malignancies and leukemia did not vary substantially among our exposure surrogate groups (i.e., those who boarded target ships after a detonation vs. those who did not, and those enlisted personnel who had an Engineering & Hull occupational specialty vs. those in other specialties).

• Participants who boarded target ships were thought to be more highly exposed than the rest of the participant group. Relative to the controls (nonparticipating comparison group), boarding participants experienced a 5.7 percent increase in all-cause mortality, RR equal to 1.057 (1.014–1.10), $p = 0.0093$, whereas the nonboarders (less exposed participant group) experienced a 4.3 percent increase (RR = 1.043 [1.015–1.073], $p = 0.0028$). Aside from all-cause mortality, risks for boarding participants did not significantly exceed those for controls for any of the disease categories, and risks relative to controls were similar for boarding and nonboarding participants. The increase in risk for all-malignancies among the participants was 2.6 percent (RR = 1.026 [0.94–1.12], $p = 0.55$) for boarders and 1 percent (RR = 1.010 [0.95–1.068], $p = 0.73$) for nonboarders. For leukemia, the increase in mortality risk for boarders was, 0.7 percent (RR = 1.007 [0.61–1.66], $p = 0.98$) and for nonboarders, 2.4 percent (RR = 1.024 [0.737–1.422], $p = 0.89$). In all cases the 95% confidence intervals

[2] All statistical tests are two-sided.

overlap, suggesting the difference between boarders and nonboarders could well be due to chance.

• Those Navy participants holding an Engineering & Hull (E&H) occupational specialty were thought to be more highly exposed to radiation than their non-E&H counterparts. However, the E&H participants had essentially the same risk of mortality from all causes as non-E&H participants (RR = 0.99 [0.95–1.038], p = .81). For all malignancies and leukemias, the rate ratios were somewhat higher, 1.051 [0.97–1.14] and 1.51 [0.94–2.44] respectively, but both could be attributed to chance (p = 0.25 and 0.088 respectively). Risk ratios for leukemia and malignancies among E&H controls showed a similar elevation relative to non-E&H controls, suggesting that a factor specifically associated with CROSSROADS was not likely to have been the cause.

These findings do not support a hypothesis that exposure to ionizing radiation was the cause of increased mortality among CROSSROADS participants. Had radiation been a significant contributor to increased risk of mortality, we should have seen significantly increased mortality due to malignancies, particularly leukemia, in participants thought to have received higher radiation doses relative to participants with lower doses and to unexposed controls. We did not observe any such effects. We note, however, that this study was neither intended not designed to be an investigation of low-level radiations effects, per se, and it should not be interpreted as such.

In comparing the findings and methods employed in this study with those of other investigations of atomic veteran mortality, we have identified a possible self-selection bias in the participant cohort: participants who died of a disease (particularly cancer) may have been more likely than healthy participants to have identified themselves to the NTPR, and hence become a part of this study. Such a bias would have resulted in an apparent increase in death rates among the participants. We do not have data with which to make a good quantitative estimate of this potential bias. However, the roster of participants is nearly complete, and mortality from all malignancies and leukemia was lower, not higher, than the increase in all-cause mortality. These factors suggest that a self-selection bias was not entirely responsible for the finding of increased all-cause mortality in study participants.

We believe that the elevated risk of all-cause mortality in CROSSROADS participants relative to a comparable military comparison group is probably the result of two factors. The first is an unidentified factor, other than radiation, associated with participation in, or presence at, the CROSSROADS test. The second is a self-selection bias within the participant roster. However, the relative contributions of these two explanations cannot be accurately determined within available resources for this project.

1

Study Rationale and Overview

RATIONALE

In July 1946, the United States conducted a test of atomic weapons code named Operation CROSSROADS. From then until the test ban treaty in 1963, the Department of Defense and earlier agencies conducted 235 nuclear detonations, involving at least 210,000 military participants—dubbed atomic veterans—in 19 test series. Fifty years later, scientists, veterans advocates, health and environmental advocates, military spokespersons, politicians, and veterans and their families debate whether and to what extent exposure to the nuclear tests affected the participants health.

The mass media showed the world pictures of fall-out covered ships and personnel. Individual participants have published vivid accounts of their experiences (e.g., Bradley 1948). Many veterans have applied to the Department of Veterans Affairs for compensation for health problems and disability they attribute to radiation exposure (*The Washington Post* and Senator Rockefeller mention more than 3,000 claims by 1984, when hearings and legislation gave impetus to this study. Studies to date (e.g., Darby 1988, 1993; Watanabe, Kang, and Dalager 1994; Robinette 1985; Campbell 1995) both government-supported and veterans-advocate designed, have added to our understanding of mortality outcomes in atomic veterans, but none has specifically addressed the mortality of CROSSROADS participants.

Congress has passed legislation and three presidents have signed three laws that address certain concerns of the atomic veterans.[3] These allow for increased priority for medical care and some loosening of record standards for compensation purposes for specific, listed health conditions.[4] In 1983, section 601 of PL 98-160 directed the Secretary of Veterans Affairs to contract with an unbiased, disinterested scientific group to study the mortality effects of atomic radiation on Operation CROSSROADS participants. The Institute of Medicine at the National Academy of Sciences was chosen.

The Medical Follow-up Agency (MFUA) of the Institute of Medicine-National Academy of Sciences presents in this report the description and findings of the mortality study it has conducted since 1986. It compared the rates and causes of death of the approximately 40,000 military personnel who were present at Operation CROSSROADS with those of a reference group of personnel not exposed to those activities. Our charge has been to answer, using the best available information on exposure and mortality outcome, the focused question: Have CROSSROADS participants had more or earlier deaths from all causes and from various specific causes than did military personnel who are alike in all respects save CROSSROADS participation? While the report discusses a somewhat broader range of questions in light of its findings, it *does not purport to answer* such questions as: Does low-level radiation cause cancer? Did the United States act appropriately, from the perspectives of medical science, environmental hazard control, and ethics, in its design and conduct of nuclear tests and follow-up activities? At the sponsor's request, we have conducted detailed verification studies to ascertain the accuracy and completeness of the CROSSROADS participant list provided to us by the Defense Nuclear Agency (DNA).[5]

In summary, this report will present data and findings about the mortality experience of CROSSROADS participants, discuss possible meanings of those findings, and suggest avenues of further study. It is outside the scope of our charter to determine what fiduciary responsibility anyone holds or should take for the health experience of those personnel. Those are questions that science alone cannot answer and this study will not address.

---

[3]Public Law 98-542, January 1984; PL 100-321, May 1988; and PL 102-578, January 1992.

[4]At the time of this report, federal statute requires the Secretary of Veterans Affairs to provide presumptive service-connected benefits to veterans with expert testimony of radiation exposure and one of the following diseases: leukemia (other than chronic lymphocytic leukemia), cancer of the thyroid, cancer of the breast, cancer of the pharynx, cancer of the esophagus, cancer of the stomach, cancer of the small intestine, cancer of the pancreas, multiple myeloma, lymphomas (except Hodgkin's disease), cancer of the bile ducts, cancer of the gall bladder, primary liver cancer (except if cirrhosis or hepatitis B is indicated), cancer of the salivary gland, and cancer of the urinary tract. VA regulations cover a few additional conditions for medical-care access.

[5]In June 1996, the Defense Nuclear Agency was renamed the Defense Special Weapons Agency.

OVERVIEW

In this study, the basic comparisons are between CROSSROADS participants and non-CROSSROADS participants. The specifics of the study plan involve choice of comparison groups and choice of outcomes to study. This study is solely a mortality study; that is, we do not consider the incidence of nonfatal or not-yet-fatal diseases in this population. The analyses are based on deaths of CROSSROADS participants and individuals in various comparison groups that occurred after the July 1946 tests through 31 December 1992.

The initial overall health outcome comparisons are:

- all-cause mortality,
- all-cancer mortality, and
- leukemia mortality.

The benefit of the first of these comparisons is its use of all the mortality information available on the participants. The drawback, too, lies in its broad scope. Our knowledge of radiation biology and earlier study findings suggested health effects on a narrower range of outcomes.

In addition to these three disease groups, which will be used to test for CROSSROADS effects, we also look, descriptively, at 44 other disease categories[6] that have been (a) identified in earlier studies of atomic veterans, (b) hypothesized to be radiogenic, (c) declared by statute or regulation to be radiogenic for purposes of federal veterans compensation programs, or (d) known to be of interest to atomic veterans.

For two reasons, we do not include other reported or hypothesized radiogenic conditions, such as ophthalmic cataract, and dermatologic, immunologic, psychiatric, and reproductive conditions. First, this study's endpoint is mortality—chosen because such data are available and definable—and most of these other conditions do not consistently result in death. Second, a recent Institute of Medicine report lays out in detail reasons for not studying adverse reproductive outcomes in atomic veterans, their spouses, and children (IOM 1995).

The participant group included all military personnel assigned to a unit and verified as being on site[7] during the official operational period of CROSSROADS: 1 July 1946 through 31 August 1946. This report compares the participants' mortality with that of three types of reference groups:

1. a military nonparticipant cohort,
2. the U.S. male population, and
3. mortality rates from other relevant published studies.

---

[6]See Chapter 10 for details.

[7]"Onsite participation" is defined in Federal Register Vol. 54, No. 118, 21 June 1989, page 26029.

A military comparison group is considered the most closely comparable to the military participants. It includes men who served in the military at the same time, in the same types of military occupations and paygrades, and in similar settings as the participants, but who did not participate in Operation CROSSROADS. Whatever the unmeasured nonradiation risk factors the participants may have carried (e.g., behavioral, such as cigarette smoking; environmental, such as living on a ship; or demographic, such as education and income), the comparison group is likely to be equivalent, reducing the opportunity for biased study results.

Comparison with the general U.S. male population is a useful adjunct to a military comparison group. Scientists and other readers of mortality studies are used to seeing U.S. rates and can weigh interpretation accordingly. A very large drawback to using U.S. population rates exists, however. The "healthy worker effect" or, in this case, the "healthy soldier effect" makes interpretation of these comparisons difficult; we discuss this in Chapter 3.

2

Other Studies of the Human Health Effects of Radiation Exposure

Human physical health effects of radiation fall along a continuum that includes immediate death, shortened lifespan due to radiogenic cancers such as leukemia, increased morbidity due to radiogenic conditions such as cataracts or nonfatal cancers, no discernible effect, and, in the view of some, beneficial physiologic response. U.S. military personnel exposed to nuclear weapons tests did not receive radiation in amounts that would be immediately lethal. The questions we addressed in this mortality study of atomic veterans concern the long-lasting, difficult-to-prove effects of lower levels of radiation that can result in increased incidence of cancer. This study looks specifically at exposed veterans. Other studies, not reviewed here (NRC 1990, UNSCEAR 1994, Shigematsu et al. 1995), have examined associations of radiation and health outcomes in groups defined by widely varying sources of radiation (for example, occupational, environmental, medical, and acts of war).

Reports from individual veterans and advocacy groups brought to attention concerns about mortality and long-term morbidity believed to be caused by the radiation exposures received during nuclear weapons testing. The leadership of the National Association of Atomic Veterans (NAAV) and Trinity Post 7-45 have collected data and testified passionately about such increased illness. The NAAV Medical Survey Data Base (see Appendix A) had information (as of 28 January 1995) on 167 deaths among the 1,263 Operation CROSSROADS participants known to NAAV. Of the 379 death certificates NAAV gathered from participants in any U.S. nuclear test (not only CROSSROADS), about 75 percent are from cancer (Campbell 1994). That appears unusually high, since national data show malignant neoplasms accounting for about 30 percent of male deaths in each 10-year age span covering deaths between ages 45 and 74. About 13 percent of years of potential life lost before age 65 is attributed to cancer deaths (NCHS 1992).

In 1976, following notice of a patient who associated his acute myelocytic leukemia with his presence at an atmospheric nuclear test, the Centers for Disease Control mounted an epidemiological study of military personnel who had attended that test—Shot SMOKY, a detonation of Operation PLUMBBOB—conducted at the Nevada test site in August 1957 (Caldwell et al. 1980, 1983). Findings of increased leukemias among participants generated concern that their health may have been adversely affected by participation in the atmospheric testing program. An extensive study of participants at five test series (chosen to represent a range of testing circumstances) was conducted by the Medical Follow-up Agency of the National Academy of Sciences (now within the Institute of Medicine) to pursue that hypothesis (Robinette et al. 1985). In 1989, the Defense Nuclear Agency informed MFUA that the data DNA had provided—and on which all MFUA analyses were based—incorrectly identified members of the participant cohort. DNA's initial estimate of the error was larger but, after detailed review, the congressional Office of Technology Assessment (OTA) estimated that approximately 15,000 names should have been but were not on the participant roster and another approximately 4,500 were wrongly included on the participant list (Gelband 1992). The total number of participants in that 1985 study was 49,148. MFUA (with support and concurrence from the OTA, the General Accounting Office, and congressional and Department of Defense staff) decided that the published study results (Robinette et al. 1985) should be withdrawn from discussion pending reexamination of the data and correction for possibly substantial errors in participant group identification. At the request of DNA, MFUA is redoing the Five Series Study with the more complete data. Results from the newer study are not expected before the end of 1997.

Other formal epidemiologic studies have not revealed distributions of rates that clearly confirm or refute radiation-caused mortality and long-term morbidity. Watanabe et al. (1995) compared military participants at Hardtack I, a 1958 U.S. test series in the Pacific, with a military comparison group. All-cause mortality (relative risk 1.10; 95% confidence interval 1.02–1.19) and digestive cancer mortality (RR 1.47; 1.06–2.04) mortality was higher among the Hardtack participants, but excess rates were not observed in deaths from all cancers, leukemia, or other hypothesized radiogenic cancers. The authors described the patterns of increased (and decreased) rates, but stopped short by neither concluding there were increased risks nor ruling them out.

Darby et al. (1993) studied mortality and cancer incidence in military participants of United Kingdom nuclear weapons tests and found no "detectable effect on expectation of life or on subsequent risk of developing cancer or other fatal diseases." Although participants had significantly higher leukemia rates than controls, the authors attribute that to an abnormally low rate among the controls rather than to a radiation-associated high rate among the participants. That both the control and the participant groups had fewer cancers than expected based on general U.K. population rates (even after controlling for social class) is presented to support that interpretation. The standardized mortality ratio (standardized to the U.K. population) for leukemias in the control groups was 0.56 for the entire follow-up period and 0.34 for the time period 2 to 25 years postexposure.

The results of this study of CROSSROADS participants and the earlier mentioned Five Series Study simultaneously under way should add more information about, and therefore a more stable understanding of, the association between nuclear test participant exposure and mortality. These studies are constructed carefully to include appropriate comparison groups and to avoid known biases (operational as well as conceptual) in the data collection and analysis, and, finally, in their interpretation.

3

Epidemiology Primer

Begin with a question such as "Does exposure X cause disease Y?" The premise of epidemiology is so deceptively simple that it can be described in two sentences:

- Scientists compare two groups of people that are alike in all ways except that one group was exposed to X and the other group was not.
- If more people in the exposed group than in the other group have the disease, Y, scientists have an epidemiologic clue that exposure X may be harmful. (Note: We have not proven that X causes Y; we have shown that in this sample X and Y occur together more often than we would have expected them to by chance.)

What, however, takes scores of technical textbooks and fuels ongoing debates are the "how to" and "what if," "buts," "on the other hands," and "howevers" that make all the difference between error-laden, error-tinged, and accurate study results. In the next few pages, we describe several known pitfalls and techniques for avoiding them. That should provide a basic background to enable non-technically oriented readers to dig into this report.

Epidemiology is the study of the distribution and determinants of disease and its effects (e.g., death) in human populations. While examining data, rather than people (as in clinical research) or animals or chemicals (as in laboratory research), epidemiologic analyses seek to understand causation. Epidemiology attempts to tease out the relationships between factors—be they characteristics of people (e.g., age, race, sex), or their work (tension-filled or relaxed, indoors or outdoors) or home (sufficient or insufficient food, shelter, and social support) environments; characteristics of potentially harmful factors (viruses, poverty, metabolic disturbances, high cholesterol, or radiation) or beneficial factors (including new medication, surgery, medical devices, health education, income, and housing); or measures of health status (mortality rates, cholesterol levels, or disease incidence). Notice that one factor can be at once a characteristic, risk factor, and outcome. A key distinction between epidemiologic and experimental data is that epidemiologic studies usually are not designed experiments with purebred animal subjects randomized to be exposed or not exposed. Rather, one makes use of exposure situations that have occurred for various reasons to learn what one can. This is essential in situations such as the study of CROSSROADS participation where a randomized design is impossible retrospectively.

It is important to understand that while epidemiology seeks to understand causal pathways, it cannot prove causation. Epidemiology uses judgment, statistics, and skepticism to reach *descriptions* and *interpretations* of relationships and associations. It is both a practical technique and an intellectual framework for considering the possibilities of causal relationships. It is the approach we have taken in this study.

Epidemiologists compare groups. The key to making sound comparisons is in choosing groups that are alike in all ways except for the matter being studied. This selection of comparison groups is where the science, mathematics, and art of good epidemiology are blended. For example, because age and sex are associated with health risks and conditions, data regarding age and sex are collected, making it possible in the analysis to either compare like age distributions and sexes or statistically adjust the data to account for known differences.

CHOICE OF COMPARISON GROUP

In studying CROSSROADS participants, comparison group options include the development of a specific control group, internal comparisons by level of exposure, and use of national statistics. Each carries useful and restrictive elements.

If, for example, one wants to study the effect of something on lung cancer, knowing what we do about cigarette smoking and lung cancer, we would want to pick two groups to compare that do not differ in smoking practices, for that difference could mask the true causal relationship we are looking to explore. In studies of military participants, it helps to use a reference group that is also military. After checking age and sex, we rest a bit more comfortably that the two groups are rather likely to be similar on a host of unmeasured characteristics—such as smoking behavior. If, however, we chanced to compare the woodwind section of the Navy band (good breathers) with an average group of smokers, we could encounter differences attributable to smoking behavior.

Closer to the concerns of this study, we would not want to compare a group exposed to nuclear test radiation with a group drawn from radiation workers. (Although if there were a few radiation workers in a much greater number of comparison group members, any possible confounding would be very diluted.)

Study results hinge on differences between the two (or more) groups compared in the study. So, choice of comparison group(s) is an extremely important task, one that has both conceptual and practical aspects. Consistent findings over hundreds of different disease-exposure inquiries demonstrate what we refer to as a "healthy worker effect." With no hypothesized harmful exposure, a cohort of workers or soldiers is *expected* to be healthier, as reflected in mortality and morbidity rates, than a general cohort. To be included in the soldier or worker cohort, the individual has to be mentally and physically functioning at or above whatever level is required for the duties of that cohort. In the extreme, those on their "deathbeds" are not hired or recruited. Furthermore, individuals are excluded from military service if they are not "fit," according to clinical and laboratory findings. Numerous studies have confirmed that this healthy worker effect is most pronounced in measurements taken close to the time of hiring (or entry into military service) but continues for decades.

Using a military comparison group addresses and avoids the healthy soldier effect but does carry other drawbacks. While government and other groups routinely gather statistics (including demographic, health, and employment descriptors) on general populations, such as U.S. males aged 45–65, data are not readily available for more finely (or even grossly) honed comparison groups in the military or elsewhere. Using a specifically designed comparison group, therefore, adds expense and time to a study. Furthermore, it increases the opportunity to introduce confounding information that could bias the findings.

Many of these difficulties can be overcome with meticulous attention to technique, innovative study designs and analytic plans, and a balanced view of what statistics do and do not say. These options are difficult to weigh for practiced scientists and no less difficult to explain to and discuss with non-technically trained readers; misunderstanding between scientist and public often occurs.

One option is to compare the group in question (for example, military personnel who participated in nuclear tests) with more than one comparison group, aiming to tease out relationships between exposure and outcome by seeing similarities and differences in those comparisons. The current CROSSROADS study is structured around a military comparison group, chosen to match on age, rank, time period, and military occupation—all available characteristics—but specifically *not* CROSSROADS test participants. Secondarily, we included statistical comparisons with the general U.S. male population.

FINE TUNING OF EXPOSED GROUP

Although "participant" vs. "nonparticipant" is an intuitively reasonable place to start analysis in this study, there are intricate details to consider. Foremost, not all "participants" received the same amount of exposure (or potential exposure, measured exposure, expected exposure, or type of exposure) as all the other participants.

We look, therefore, for some way(s) of measuring the amount of exposure and then characterizing individuals in relation to their known (or expected or hypothesized) dose (amount of exposure). Otherwise, if only a few of the participants were exposed, any effect (on cancer mortality, for example) would be diluted because most of the "exposed" were actually "not exposed" (or minimally exposed) and would not reflect the exposure-disease association. No difference would be observed and we would not know whether that meant there was indeed no difference or the comparison groups were identified in ways in which a real difference could not be observed.

Because adequate direct exposure measurements are not always available, researchers attempt to develop surrogate measures of exposure. In this study we pursued data from actual dosimetry measurements made at the time of the nuclear tests, recalculations done to address the known incompleteness of those measures, self-reports of participants, and coherent assumptions based on knowledge of radiation physics, troop logistics, on-site reportage, logs, and documents as well as logic.

CONFOUNDERS

It will come as no surprise that some characteristics—such as age and sex—are associated with numerous measures of health status. They are, also, associated with military experience in general and CROSSROADS participation in particular. These are likely confounders (things that confuse a straightforward comparison), because they are characteristics associated with both the outcome and the putative causative element under study. While a military comparison group based on broad categories of age, sex, similar unit assignment, and military rank provides some assurance of comparability, differences are still likely to exist. When we know what the confounders are *and* we can measure them, we can take them into account in the statistical analysis. Careful choice of comparison groups can help to limit the effect of unknown confounders. Chapters 10 and 11 of this report describe the design and analytic steps we took to control for potential confounding.

Examples of characteristics that frequently confound exposure-disease associations include age, race, sex, socioeconomic status, occupation, and various behaviors, such as alcohol and tobacco use. In specific studies investigators may hypothesize potential confounders such as ethnicity; military service-related exposures, including sunlight, altitude, preventive and therapeutic attention to infectious disease as well as the diseases themselves; and other risks based on lifestyle, geography, and postmilitary careers.

DATA COLLECTION

Once researchers have chosen the groups to study, avoiding the pitfalls—or at least, recognizing and measuring them as best as possible for later adjustment, they face a new set of problems during the planning and conduct of data collection. If you plan to get information directly from the subject, you need to do all you can to find all subjects, regardless of their being in the case/participant or control/comparison group and regardless of the outcome under study. If you are getting information from records, you need to get records for all subjects, again regardless of their being in the case/participant or control/comparison group and regardless of the outcome under study.

For example, if you are attempting to get information from subjects themselves and want to find out mortality rates and gather information by phone, *you will not find anyone to be dead.* Conversely, if you look only at death certificates, *you will not find anyone alive.* These somewhat tongue-in-cheek extremes are easy to avoid; the shades of gray around and between them, however, are often stumbling blocks in data collection and then analysis and interpretation. The reasons are that there are biases in record systems: not all records have an equal likelihood of being retrieved. For example, in looking at hospital records, specific cases involved in lawsuits may be in the general counsel's office and not in the clinic's file, where they would normally be found. There are also mundane reasons for all data not being equally available: records can be lost or destroyed, intentionally or unintentionally, by flood or fire, as in the case of veterans' records at the National Personnel Records Center in St. Louis (see Chapter 7). Note that bias does not necessarily mean prejudicial treatment, but would include any process that systematically treats one set of records differently than another.

To minimize possible biases, a number of general rules and protocols have evolved to guide researchers—regardless of participant or comparison group and regardless of likely outcome. These protocols include developing an understanding of all data sources and how they may be expected to affect data distributions and establishing clear decision rules. A summary list of rules could include:

- ensuring that there is an equal likelihood of finding records of people in each group; if a source of data is available for only one group, do not use it.
- being aware of biases built into record systems. There are potentially many of these: people with illness are more likely to seek care; veterans with

lower incomes or service-connected disabilities are more likely to seek VA care; care-seeking behavior varies over time (for example, as VA benefits change); medical record technologies change; whether patients or family members have concerns about benefits or suspicions of causation could influence whether they notify the recordkeeping agency; data may be missing due to circumstances beyond human control, such as a fire destroying paper files; and data accuracy is associated with level of ascertainment, such as completeness of fact-of-death, date-of-death, or cause-of-death information.

• using a firm cut-off date for the follow-up period. It is necessary to treat participants and comparisons equally when it comes to data collection, follow-up, and maintenance. The decisions made should be definable. Researchers should examine—according to biologic, logistical, and cost implications—choices involving latency periods, cohort age, or pending compensation questions. Once cut-offs are chosen, it is best to recognize and honor the choice (although it may seem arbitrary in practice).

• recognizing that raw numbers offer different information than do rates or proportions. The latter include a context for interpreting the importance of the raw number. While reporting the number of people dead is often informative, it is insufficient to use *percentages* without first identifying a conceptually acceptable denominator and then using the *entire* denominator in any calculation. For example, when examining constructs such as "average age at death," one should account for the amount of time available for observations since the average will change over time as larger proportions of the sample die. For example, let's follow the mortality experience of a hypothetical sixth-grade class of 25 students in 1923. Looking at them in 1925, after one 13-year-old died in a motor vehicle accident, we would see an average age at death of 13 years. If no one else in that class were to die over the next 15 years, then, in 1940, the average age at death would still be 13 because all members of the cohort who had died (in this case one person) did so at age 13. By 1975 (the original children would now be about 61 years old), perhaps another 10 had died; the average age at death would be higher than 13, but necessarily lower than 61. The average would depend on when the deaths occurred within that period. The average age of death calculated at any point in time is the average of the ages at death for all members deceased by that point in time. The average will change over time as more deaths are added into the calculations. The average does not reflect the total mortality experience of the group until *all* members have died. Statistical techniques have been developed to even out such things, so that numbers can be compared meaningfully.

These comments show the bridges among data collection, reporting, and analysis. In the following sections, we continue with analysis issues.

INTERPRETING DATA FINDINGS

Let us say that comparison groups were chosen appropriately, unbiased data collected, and one group has more disease than the other. Epidemiology provides for the use of judgment in considering whether a numerical relationship might reflect a causal one. The criteria of causal judgment—which have been stated in many contexts—involve two broad considerations: Are the exposure and the outcome *associated*? Does that association *make sense*, based on biological as well as other physical, historical, and study design factors?

Epidemiology studies are designed to describe numerical associations between factors (risks, treatments, outcomes). In interpreting the results we look at characteristics of those associations. Evidence supporting a causal association mounts if the association is consistent (observed in a variety of studies addressing the same type of exposure in different circumstances), strong (e.g., with high relative risk ratios), and specific. Statistics serve as a tool to quantify the strength of associations relative to random background fluctuations, which are more likely to be observed the smaller the sample considered. Through mathematical theory and centuries of data analysis, statisticians have derived (and continue to derive) methods to deal with multiple comparisons, effects of misclassification, inferences from samples, and combining data from diverse (but not too diverse) studies.

Vital to the epidemiologist's examination of data are the issues of statistical measures and variability. Starting with a sample of people, we generate statistical measures (or statistics, for short) that summarize some important information collected on them (e.g., death rates). Variability enters the picture when we take a particular sample, because the statistics we generate for that particular sample will be specific to that sample; a different sample would generate different statistics because the individuals in one sample are not the same as in the other. Yet, if a sample has been selected essentially at random and something is known or assumed about the distribution of the statistics generated from that particular sample, then we can make some general statements about the variability of those statistics.

Typically, we characterize a particular statistical measure's variability by quantifying how much it would vary just by taking different samples and recalculating that same statistic. In general, it turns out that the larger the sample, the smaller the variability. It is customary to calculate two limits, called the lower and upper 95 percent confidence limits, that have the property that if we repeatedly drew samples and recalculated the statistic, these different values would lie between the upper and lower confidence limits 95 times out of 100. The interval between the upper and lower confidence limits is thus called a 95 percent confidence interval. The wider the confidence interval, the more variability there is in the statistic.

It is frequently of interest to know what the variability of a statistic is because it affects its interpretation. If the mortality rates of participants and controls are equal, for example, then the ratio of these two rates (the rate ratio) should be 1.0. However, there is inherent variability in this rate ratio statistic, so that we want to calculate its 95 percent confidence interval. If the ratio is only slightly more than or less than 1.0, for example, by an amount that lies within the confidence interval, we customarily conclude that this small deviation from 1.0 could be attributed to inherent variability (chance), such as that which comes from selecting different samples. On the other hand, if the confidence interval for the rate ratio does not include 1.0, its value is not attributed to chance and it is considered statistically significant.

Another way to determine whether a particular statistic (let us stick to rate ratios) is bigger or smaller than 1.0 is to perform a statistical test. A statistical test is a more formal statistical procedure that computes a statistic under the assumption that some null hypothesis is true. A typical null hypothesis might be: there is *no* difference in mortality rate between group A and group B (in other words, the rate ratio is equal to 1.0). If the statistic is "unusual," then the null hypothesis is rejected. The measure of "unusual" is called a p-value. Customarily, a p value of less than 0.05 is considered "unusual." For example, take the above null hypotheses of no difference between mortality rates in groups A and B; i.e, the rate ratio is 1.0. If observed data yield an actual rate ratio of 1.5, for instance, and an associated test statistic with a p-value less than 0.05, then we reject the null hypothesis and conclude that such a high risk ratio is unlikely (only 5 times out of 100) to be due to chance.

Finally, we need to examine a little more what "unlikely to be due to chance" means in a larger context. By custom, a value is called statistically significant if the operation of chance will produce such a value only about 5 times in 100. However, just as in the case of repeated samples, repeated analyses of different data (for example, death rates due to cancer, to heart disease, to respiratory disease, etc.), every one involving a statistical test will carry an individual 5 percent risk of labeling a statistic significant when its increased or decreased value was actually due to chance.

Moreover, if we do many such analyses, that 5 percent risk for each one mounts up. For example, if one does 20 statistical tests of rate ratios, it is quite likely that there will be at least one rate ratio labeled statistically significant just by the operation of chance. This analytic problem is known as the multiple comparisons problem.

Because the greater the number of statistical tests, the more findings are labeled statistically significant due to chance, efforts are made to limit the number of statistical tests. This is usually done by specifying in advance a relatively small number of tests, directed at a limited number of research questions. Nevertheless, there are also times—for example, when one is interested in completely describing all the data, say, looking at a complete list of causes of death, whether or not one suspects that any of these rates are elevated—when many independent tests are made. In these situations, it is especially important to keep in mind the possibility that statistically significant rate ratios may be labeled so merely due to chance.

At the same time, one must consider that a true association may fail to test as statistically significant by chance or because of lack of statistical power. The power of a study to detect a real association (if there were one) depends on sample size, the incidence of the outcome in the absence of exposure, and the strength of association between the exposure and the outcome.

In considering whether an observed association makes sense causally, epidemiologists consider the temporal relationship between the factors (e.g., if described appropriately, an outcome cannot precede a cause), the biologic plausibility of the association, and its coherence with a range of other related knowledge (radiation biology, for example). No one of these factors is necessarily sufficient to prove causation. In fact, causation cannot actually be proven; it can only be supported (weakly or strongly) or contradicted (weakly or strongly).

Epidemiology uses numbers, going to extreme lengths at times to "split hairs" and "search under rocks," yet relies on judgment for interpretation. It is hoped that the considered judgments of epidemiologists will be useful to the judgment of clinicians in making treatment decisions and of policymakers in making legislation and regulatory and procedural decisions.

EPIDEMIOLOGY SUMMARY RELATED TO THIS STUDY

This is a report of a retrospective cohort study comparing military participants in CROSSROADS with military nonparticipants who are similar in age, rank-rating, military occupation, time frame of service, and sex. To more accurately measure exposure, we developed and used criteria for those participants most likely to have been more highly exposed. The study design calls for tight controls on the selection process for assignment to participant or comparison groups, data access, and data follow-up.

The endpoints considered are mortality rates. Specific causes of death were chosen based on understanding of disease process and *a priori* expectations based on knowledge and suspicion of radiation effects.

This study will *not* say whether Private Rogers, Rodriguez, or Rosenthal died of cancer because of Operation CROSSROADS. It *may* be able to say that the rate of cancer among all CROSSROADS participants was—or was not—different from the rate of cancer among comparable nonparticipants. Whether associations are reported with relative surety or uncertainty depends on the data themselves and on statistical techniques for sifting the wheat from the chaff. If this were easy, we would not still be studying and arguing about radiation effects.

The Medical Follow-up Agency of the Institute of Medicine, National Academy of Sciences, conducted the study, relying, as necessary, on records maintained by government and private groups. MFUA is itself "disinterested" in that it stands to neither lose nor gain from its findings in this study: it will neither receive nor be denied compensation, nor will it be held fiscally or programmatically responsible for such compensation or related care. Because this study (not unlike many other studies of human suffering and possible blame and responsibility) has an historical overlay of tremendous emotion and distrust, we must be especially careful to follow generally accepted ground rules for valid studies and to describe openly our rationale for various decisions throughout.

4

Description of Operation CROSSROADS

The Defense Nuclear Agency (DNA) has produced detailed documents about each nuclear test series. DNA Report 6032F (1984) describes activities during Operation CROSSROADS, including primary documents such as ship logs. DNA's public affairs office issued a two-page fact sheet on CROSSROADS, dated 5 April 1984, from which the following description draws heavily.

In July 1946, the U.S. military conducted Operation CROSSROADS to determine, in a controlled way, "the effects of nuclear weapons on ships, equipment, and material." This first nuclear weapon test series at the Pacific Proving Grounds consisted of two detonations, ABLE (detonated at an altitude of 520 feet) and BAKER (detonated 90 feet under water), each with a yield of approximately 23 kilotons.[8]

More than 90 vessels were positioned as the target fleet, while approximately 150 other ships were used to transport and house personnel and accommodate technical stations, such as laboratories and workshops. Approximately 42,000 men[9] participated on site at some time during the CROSSROADS official operational period (1 July through 31 August 1946).

[8]The Hiroshima bomb was 15 kilotons.

[9]Consonant with military practice in the 1940s, there were not many women involved in naval ship-based operations. DNA data indicate a few women (perhaps 25) on board. We include them in analyses but have chosen to use male comparison mortality rates.

Before each detonation, all participants were evacuated from target vessels and the Bikini Atoll to locations at least 10 nautical miles away.

Shot ABLE was released from the air on 1 July 1946, detonating about 1750 feet off target and sinking five ships. Most surviving target ships were reboarded within 24 hours. Activities in preparation for BAKER, including vessel inspection, instrument recovery, and remooring, continued on schedule.

On 25 July 1946, the detonation of BAKER created such pressure under water that huge splashes from the bottom of the lagoon sprayed radioactive water and debris over most of the target fleet. This limited the possible activities on target ships, such as physical inspections or pickup of the recorder and measurement devices. In early August, efforts began to decontaminate the fleet by intensive washing of ship surfaces; all boarding parties were accompanied by radiological monitors, who were responsible for identifying and limiting exposure to radiation. DNA describes radiological supervision in its fact sheet (1984):

> All CROSSROADS operations were undertaken under radiological supervision intended to keep personnel from being exposed to more than 0.1 roentgen per day. At the time, this was considered to be an amount of radiation that could be tolerated for long periods without any harmful effects on health.
>
> Radiological supervision included predicting areas of possible danger, providing trained personnel equipped with radiation survey instruments to act as guides during operations involving potential exposure, and elaboration of rules and regulations governing conduct in these operations. Personnel were removed for one or more days from areas and activities of possible exposure if their badges showed more than 0.1 R/day exposure
>
> About 15 percent of the JTF 1 personnel was issued at least one of the 18,875 film-badge dosimeters during CROSSROADS. Approximately 6,596 personnel were on islands or ships that had no potential for radiation exposure. Personnel anticipated to be at greatest radiological risk were badged, and a percentage of each group working in less contaminated areas was badged. The maximum accumulated exposure recorded (was 3.72 R received by) a radiation safety monitor[ing person].

This report discusses radiation measurement and dosimetry at length in Chapter 8.

Support ships were soon registering contamination, arising from radioactive marine growth on hulls and radioactive water being piped through ships' systems. Between 10 August and the end of September 1946, target ships were towed to Kwajalein Atoll, where the water was uncontaminated, for ammunition off-loading and further work.

Most target vessels were eventually sunk in the area, but 12 ships were reboarded by their crews and sailed to the U.S., and others were towed to the U.S. and Hawaii for radiological inspection. Before returning to the fleet, support ships had to receive radiological clearance; if necessary, they underwent decontamination.

DNA designates the period 1 July through 31 August 1946 as Operation CROSSROADS, adding the 6-month period 1 September 1946 through 28 February 1947 as the "post-CROSSROADS" period. The period after that, however, despite ongoing work in Navy yards and in the atoll on contaminated ships, is officially considered neither the CROSSROADS nor post-CROSSROADS period.

5

Data Sources for the CROSSROADS Study

The next part of this report describes procedures of the study in detail, referring frequently to numerous documents, records, and sources with which many readers will not be familiar. Here, therefore, we briefly enumerate the sources and describe their general limitations and assets.

Study staff, as well as Department of Defense (DoD) staff and contractors, made strenuous attempts to identify the existence of any relevant records, to acquire those records, and to corroborate information from multiple sources. Data related to personnel movements, radiation exposure, and vital status relevant to this study proved to be dispersed across the nation in cartons, computers, and file cabinets under the authority of many federal, state, and local agencies.

The following federal agencies and facilities maintain collections that the study staff used: DoD (not organized as such during the time of CROSSROADS), including the Navy, Army, Air Force, and Marines, and the Defense Nuclear Agency's Nuclear Test Personnel Review; the Department of Veterans Affairs, including its benefit and health organizations; the Department of Health and Human Services, including the Health Care Financing Administration and the National Center for Health Statistics, which maintains the National Death Index; and the National Archives and Records Administration's National Personnel Records Center, Federal Archives Records Centers, and Office of the National Archives. Central office and regionally maintained records were reviewed by study staff, agency staff, and contractors.

We requested cause-of-death information directly from state (and some municipal) vital statistics offices.[10]

Differences in record ownership affect the rules that apply to the use of data. Ease or difficulty with access, privacy, fees, time frames, and definitions (conceptual and operational) were all factors in determining collection of the data upon which this report is based. Furthermore, among the federal agencies and private sources pursued, there are different interests (some overlapping, some in seeming conflict) behind the collection of data. These purposes might include understanding science, assuring that the government honors reasonable claims for compensation, learning lessons for application to future public policy decisions, cost accounting, advocacy support (legislative, regulatory, and emotional), and assigning responsibility for past decisions and their consequences.

The completeness and accuracy of the various data collections vary widely, as does the quality of the data themselves. Certain data may be perfect for their intended purpose but not otherwise useful. Other data—such as those which we worked to retrieve for this study—may have fortuitous uses other than those for which they were collected. Trade-offs exist in data sources: accurate but limited in time frame or population considered; broadly relevant but of variable and difficult-to-judge accuracy; and relevant but lacking linked information to other lifetime experiences that might affect health status. Some sources are based on information about individuals (e.g., military personnel records), some on direct measurement (e.g., radiation dose measurements), and others on expert-derived best estimates (dose reconstructions).

Among those sources viewed were handwritten paper logs, microfilm/fiche, computer files, medical records, work orders, transport orders, memoirs,

---

[10]For sending us death certificate information, we thank government personnel in Alabama, Alaska, Arizona, Arkansas, California, Colorado, Connecticut, Delaware, the District of Columbia, Florida, Georgia, Hawaii, Idaho, Illinois, Indiana, Iowa, Kansas, Kentucky, Louisiana, Maine, Maryland, Michigan, Minnesota, Mississippi, Missouri, Nevada, New Hampshire, New Jersey, New Mexico, New York, North Carolina, Ohio, Oklahoma, Oregon, Pennsylvania, Puerto Rico, Rhode Island, South Carolina, South Dakota, Tennessee, Texas, Utah, Virginia, Washington, West Virginia, and Wisconsin. In the conduct of this study, individually identified data have been safeguarded in accordance with the Privacy Act; death certificates will be destroyed one year from publication the of CROSSROADS study manuscripts.

interoffice memoranda, testimony, secondary compilations of primary sources, letters from spouses, death certificates, burial notices, film badge records, computer programs, and benefits and compensation claims.

While any one type or source of data may be biased; taken together, these biases sometimes offset each other, at least partially. And, when independent sources corroborate specific facts, confidence in the accuracy of the information increases.

6

The Participant Cohort

The basic comparison is between groups of military personnel: those who participated in Operation CROSSROADS and a comparison cohort chosen from among those who did not. In this section we describe the process of participant cohort selection in detail, since misclassification in participant selection would decrease the likelihood of observing any exposure-outcome association that might exist.

The Defense Nuclear Agency (DNA) defined "participation" according to a 1989 announcement in the *Federal Register,*[11] to include official military

---

[11]Federal Register Vol. 54, No 118, Wednesday, June 21, 1989, Rules and Regulations, p. 26029.

"(4) For purposes of this section:

(i) The term 'radiation-exposed veteran' means a veteran who, while serving on active duty, participated in a radiation-risk activity.

(ii) The term 'radiation-risk activity' means:

(A) Onsite participation in a test involving the atmospheric detonation of a nuclear device by the United States. . . .

(iii) The term 'atmospheric detonation' includes underwater nuclear detonations.

(iv) The term 'onsite participation' means:

(A) During the official operational period of an atmospheric nuclear test, presence at the test site, or performance of official military duties in connection with ships, aircraft or other equipment used in direct support of the nuclear test.

(B) During the six month period following the official operational period of an atmospheric nuclear test, presence at the test site or other test staging area to perform official military duties in connection with completion of projects related to the nuclear test including decontamination of equipment used during the nuclear test.

activities onsite between 1 July 1946 and 31 August 1946 or involving materiel used at the tests. It provided rosters of CROSSROADS participants to the Medical Follow-up Agency (MFUA) in two stages: an initial file in 1986 and the final file in 1994.

When this study was begun, each military service maintained its own Nuclear Test Personnel Review (NTPR) activity, responsible, among other things, for identifying veterans involved in the above-ground nuclear test program. In 1986, Navy and Army NTPR offices provided data to MFUA for approximately 40,500 alleged nonduplicate participants. Air Corps personnel were covered by Army records at that time; the Navy provided Marine Corps records.

In 1992, work was interrupted on this project.[12] By the time MFUA resumed the study in 1994, DNA had consolidated the service-based NTPR teams into a single effort. DNA, via the consolidated NTPR, performed extensive data clean-up efforts to bring participant data from different branches into a common format; to update, verify, and correct data; and to create a unique identifier (heretofore nonexistent) for each record. In August 1994, DNA supplied MFUA with that updated participant list. It is the basis of the current study.

For both the 1986 file and the 1994 file, DNA identified the ships that participated at Bikini Atoll during the CROSSROADS operational period. Individuals assigned to those ships at that time plus some individuals serving at Kwajalein and Enewetak islands to support CROSSROADS were identified using the following data sources: "service personnel records, unit diaries, ship deck logs, ship/unit muster rolls, ship/unit officer lists, unit histories, morning reports, and operation participant listings."[13] Data items sought were name, rank, and service number, although date and place of birth were also noted in the 1986 file. The quality of the various identifiers varied; other identifiers, such as Social Security Number, were noted when available.

A participant cohort numbering 42,548 was developed across all military branches, using the individuals identified in the 1994 file; data items for those individuals were augmented with 1986 information as appropriate.

(C) Service as a member of the garrison or maintenance forces on Eniwetok during the periods June 21, 1951 through July 1, 1952, August 7, 1956 through August 7, 1957 or November 1, 1958 through April 30, 1959.

(D) Assignment to official military duties at Naval Shipyards involving the decontamination of ships that participated in Operation Crossroads.

(v) The term 'operational period' means: . . .

(B) For operation CROSSROADS the period July 1, 1946 through August 31, 1946. (Authority 38 U.S.C. 312)"

[12]Circumstances—including the illness and death of the principal investigator, Dr. Dennis Robinette and federal funding shortages—caused this study to be put on hold.

[13]DNA memorandum dated 11 July 1994 (see Appendix B).

It is important to realize that some of the individuals in the roster of atomic veterans may have identified themselves to DNA and subsequently become enrolled in the NTPR program as valid participants when their involvement with atomic testing had been verified. We refer to this in our discussion of the findings of this study (Chapter 11).

INDEPENDENT VERIFICATION OF PARTICIPANT COHORT

To examine the validity of the ongoing participant ascertainment process, MFUA staff then worked to characterize the variation between the initial 1986 and final 1994 files. Based on the verification process that we describe in detail in Appendix E, we estimate that approximately 2 to 4 percent of the individuals included in the 1994 participant cohort were not, in fact, participants.

Two non-DNA sources were sought to enable MFUA to estimate an independent assessment of DNA's false negative (missing actual participants) rate. The National Association of Atomic Veterans (NAAV) has run mail-in surveys (Appendix A) to develop a list of radiation-exposed veterans; it provided this list to MFUA. Also, MFUA placed announcements in large-circulation veterans' magazines, requesting "atomic veterans" to write in and identify themselves. Details of the work comparing the DNA, NAAV, and magazine write-in groups are presented in Appendix E. Overall, the matching of names indicated a high degree of agreement and, therefore, confidence in using the DNA cohort.

EXCLUSION OF "POST-CROSSROADS" PARTICIPANTS

To maintain clarity of cohort definition, this study does not include so-called "post-CROSSROADS" participants, those military personnel who arrived in the designated area after the formal cut-off date of the operation but within the six-month period 1 September 1946 through 28 February 1947.

CROSSROADS PARTICIPANTS WHO PARTICIPATED IN OTHER NUCLEAR TESTS

This report on the CROSSROADS test uses "participation" status as a general proxy for exposure (see expanded discussion in Chapter 8). Some CROSSROADS participants also attended nuclear tests other than CROSSROADS (Table 6-1). For perspective, we present the distribution of CROSSROADS participants by their presence at additional atomic tests.

TABLE 6-1. Distribution of Participation in Nuclear Test Series

Number of Nuclear Test Series in which Person Participated	CROSSROADS Participants	
	Number	Percent
CROSSROADS only	38,203	89.8
CROSSROADS plus 1 other	3,913	9.2
CROSSROADS plus 2 others	333	0.8
CROSSROADS plus 3 others	38	0.1
CROSSROADS plus 4 others	14	0.03
CROSSROADS plus 5 others	8	0.02
CROSSROADS plus 6 others	10	0.02
CROSSROADS plus 7 others	1	0.002
CROSSROADS plus 8 others	3	0.007
CROSSROADS plus 9 others	1	0.002
CROSSROADS plus 10 others	1	0.002
CROSSROADS plus 11 others	1	0.002
Total	42,526*	~100

*This count includes all participants, not only Navy personnel.

Note that 90 percent (n = 38,203) of CROSSROADS participants did not participate in any other military nuclear test. Of the remaining 10 percent (n = 4,323) who did, most (90.5 percent) were in only one other test (with almost half of those qualifying only by their inclusion in post-CROSSROADS activities, which we consider a separate test series for classification purposes).

PRIMARY ANALYSIS—NAVY PERSONNEL ONLY

The participant cohort was 91 percent Navy personnel. Because Navy records were the most complete (as will be discussed in Chapter 9), primary analyses for this report are limited to the 38,662 participating Navy personnel.

EXCLUSIVITY OF PARTICIPANT AND COMPARISON COHORTS

The comparison roster was checked against the participant roster. The 205 Navy individuals appearing on both were deleted from the control roster for this report's analyses.

7

The Comparison Cohort

A significant feature of the design of this study of Operation CROSSROADS mortality is the inclusion of a military comparison cohort. One of the criticisms of MFUA's earlier study of nuclear weapons test participants was its lack of a control group (GAO 1992). While the CROSSROADS study does compare participant mortality with that of the U.S. general population, the study has assembled, at significant cost, a separate control group from military unit and individual records. The comparison of participant death rates with rates for comparable controls should eliminate the risk of bias introduced by the "healthy soldier effect."[14]

COMPARISON COHORT SELECTION

Navy and Shipboard Marines

The Defense Nuclear Agency (DNA) provided lists of potential control units[15] to the Medical Follow-up Agency (MFUA). For Navy controls, initial plans called for selecting a control ship to pair with each participant ship.

---

[14]See discussion in Chapter 3.

[15]In the Navy, a "unit" is usually a ship (so that all personnel assigned to a particular ship would be in one unit associated with the ship's name). Exceptions occur, especially during special non-combat procedures. Examples of unit assignment could then include "RADSAFE" or "JTF" (joint task force). Army units are more frequently based on function, such as artillery or infantry.

Pairing criteria included type of ship (i.e., destroyer, cruiser, tender), Pacific location, and service near to the time of CROSSROADS.

The initial selection plan was amended twice. First, because CROSSROADS occurred in the summer of 1946, well after demobilization efforts had gotten under way following World War II, ships in the Atlantic were chosen when it was impossible to find sufficient ships of a given type in the Pacific. Second, because selected control ships did not always supply sufficient numbers of personnel for the comparison cohort to match the desired rating distribution, additional control ships were selected to provide supplements. The additional ships maintain the type of ship choice initially derived from the to-be-matched participant ship.

As discussed above, DNA supplied MFUA with lists of potential control ships; MFUA selected actual control ships from those lists. To identify the enlisted men on these ships, microfilmed muster rolls were obtained from the National Archives. Each muster roll of a Navy ship from the CROSSROADS era provides, for a given date, the complete list in alphabetical order of enlisted personnel on board that particular ship, showing name, service number, and rank/rating (for example, "MM1" is machinist mate, first class).

We selected Navy enlisted controls in such a way that they would have the same rating distribution as participants and would have served on the same types of ships. Before keying individual control names, MFUA developed a distribution of ranks and ratings (based on distribution within participant units) required from each control ship to create a balanced comparison cohort. A muster roll was selected for a control ship, and once the ship identifying information was entered into the computer, the program randomly selected a letter of the alphabet at which keying of the muster roll data for that ship was begun. As each individual rank and rating was entered, it was compared to the distribution of participant ranks and ratings for a specific ship or ship type. If a particular category had not already been filled, the keyer was allowed to enter the corresponding name and military service number. As more names were entered, more rank-rating categories were filled up, and the program accepted fewer names. Although the original software was programmed to match each individual's participant ship to a single control ship, it was later modified to match the type of participant ship to the type of control ship (e.g., submarine to submarine, destroyer to destroyer, etc.). The identification of control officers relied on a different source—deck logs—because Navy officers are not routinely listed on muster rolls.

Marine controls were selected, by and large, in the same way as Navy controls, starting from ship muster rolls. Because 52 percent had missing military service numbers (MSN), the Marine Corps Stat list was searched for MSN; the majority of missing numbers were found. Also, there was no random alphabetical starting point for keying and no range checks on keyed data because, for each selected control unit, the entire list was keyed.

Army and Army Air Corps

The assembly of the Army and Army Air Corps control rosters was somewhat more complicated than that for Navy and Marines. First, although data on rank were available, there was no information on individual military occupational specialties readily at hand. In addition, the choice of Army and Army Air Corps units was less straightforward than for Navy units, because there were many more types of Army units than there were types of ships. Most important, however, was the part played by a fire at the National Personnel Records Center (NPRC) in St. Louis.

In 1973, a fire at NPRC (Stender 1974) destroyed some 80 percent of Army and Air Force personnel records from World War I through the Korean Conflict. After the fire, NPRC created a computerized registry, in part to index which military personnel records were reconstructed from fragments of burned records and which only suffered water damage and subsequently were refiled. The postfire protocol calls for all newly accessioned records to be indexed in the registry. The registry file is thus an index to the location of military medical and personnel records at NPRC. It contains information on approximately 23 million veterans. Because all selected controls were to have their military personnel records abstracted, the NPRC registry was used to obtain unburned records for controls. The 80 percent loss of records meant that there was a need to oversample from Army and Army Air Corps unit records—by roughly a factor of five—to obtain sufficient potential controls to ensure finding a control with an unburned record. Because of this oversampling strategy, the data entry software for Army and Army Air Corps records did not keep a count of each rank category; for each control unit selected, the entire unit roster was keyed.

The processing of Navy muster rolls and Army unit rosters began in October 1988 and continued through January 1990. A total of 57,734 control records were keyed, allowing for the oversampling of Army controls.

MILITARY PERSONNEL RECORDS

It was necessary to locate (using military service number) and abstract the military personnel record for each selected control individual to obtain the necessary information for a mortality analysis. Data abstracted included full name; branch of service; additional military service numbers; date, place and state of birth; place of entry onto active duty; race; rank at separation; date of separation; and whether records had been sent to the VA.

Due to blurred or unreadable microfilm, many of the service numbers keyed from the muster rolls did not correspond to records available on known military personnel. Thus, it was necessary to go to an independent source, the VA Master Index, to verify identification data. The VA Master Index (VAMI), now a large microfilm file, originally consisted of some tens of millions of 3 × 5 cards, one card for each veteran beneficiary. Each 3 × 5 card in VAMI, which was maintained in active use through the early 1970s, contains identifying and VA benefits data for an individually identified veteran. When a muster roll entry could not be matched to an available record folder, an attempt was made to locate the corresponding 3 × 5 card in VAMI and to verify correct identifying data, such as name and MSN. At the same time, additional data, if available, were also recorded: for example, VA claim number or date of death. Using these new identification data, another attempt was then made to find a record folder. Finally, despite the deliberate oversampling of Army and Army Air Corps controls, it was not always possible to find enough unburned records for men of a particular rank, and partially burned records were occasionally ordered. A total of 40,354 military personnel records were abstracted.

ADDITIONAL CONTROLS

In 1989, DNA notified MFUA that the DNA list of CROSSROADS participants reflected substantial numbers of individuals who should not be on the list and omitted many who should be on the list.[16] The final participant roster used in this study is about 2,500 individuals larger than the 1986 list on which control selection was based. The balance of ranks and ratings in ship types in the existing control pool and the participant cohort were compared and noted to be similar. Since the analysis did not involve pairwise comparisons, we determined that additional controls would not be required.

[16]See Chapter 2 of this report.

8

Exposure Definition, Measurement, and Verification

INTRODUCTION

Chapter 6 describes at length how the participant cohort was defined and assembled for this study. Status as an Operation CROSSROADS participant is the most reliable (though broad) measure of exposure and, therefore, the core variable on which to compare groups in this study. The participant vs. nonparticipant (comparison group) dichotomy provides the largest group of people to study, size being important when considering rare outcomes such as leukemia. Using participant status to represent *exposure,* in this case exposure to an atmospheric nuclear test (including ionizing radiation and possibly other environmental factors) has many limitations for use in an epidemiologic study. The fact of participant status does not provide individual-level information regarding:

- differences in potential radiation exposure among participants (see note 1 for the *Federal Register's* definition of participation);
- potential for internal as well as external radiation exposure;
- extent, if any, of participation (and, therefore, potential exposure) in test series other than CROSSROADS;
- exposure to other ill-defined environmental or occupational factors, either related to or independent of nuclear test participation (for example, post-

CROSSROADS employment as a radiological technician or a radiation worker in the nuclear power industry).

Therefore, while retaining as basic the participant vs. nonparticipant comparison, we attempted to develop more refined measures of radiation exposure. After providing a historical backdrop to the dosimetry issues, this chapter describes the approaches we considered, details about the validity of those options, and the decisions upon which we base our analyses.

DOSIMETRY BACKGROUND

The National Research Council's 1985 study (Robinette et al. 1985) used dose data provided by the Defense Nuclear Agency's (DNA) Nuclear Test Personnel Review program, which attempted to assign to each individual participant a valid estimate of the radiation dose he had received (DNA 1984). Therefore, the initial plans for the Medical Follow-up Agency (MFUA) study of CROSSROADS participants reported here included the use of these individual dose assignments.

Later, a committee of another MFUA nuclear test exposure project[17] reviewed the DNA dosimetry estimating procedures and results and issued a letter report (IOM 1995), stating that the dosimetry estimates were not appropriate for dose response analyses used in epidemiologic studies. The CROSSROADS committee and staff, based on that letter report and their own judgment, decided not to use the individual dose data in this study. We set out to explore other exposure proxies, determining how they correlated with each other and with the DNA-assigned individual dose estimates.

Definition of Potential Surrogate Dose Groups

We consider four broad ways in which to categorize exposure:

1. DNA-assigned doses,
2. participant status,
3. target ship boarding status, and
4. Engineering & Hull specialty status

Each of these adds intuitive interpretive possibilities to the analysis, while at the same time involving a wide range of validity and precision. We discuss each in turn, offering definitions, advantages, and both practical and theoretical drawbacks to use as a dose surrogate.

[17]Committee to Study the Mortality of Military Personnel Present at Atmospheric Tests of Nuclear Weapons (also known as the Five Series committee); committee chair, Clark W. Heath, Jr., M.D.; dosimetry working group chair, John Till, Ph.D.

DNA-Provided Dose Estimates

Overall

The Nuclear Test Personnel Review (NTPR) database contains a dose assignment for each participant derived, in most cases, by reconstruction based on duty assignments. In a small percentage of cases, the assigned dose is based on one or more film badges worn by the participant or on a film badge worn by another participant in the same unit at CROSSROADS (cohort badging).

Ideally, exposure measurements would be (a) individual-specific; (b) recorded by time, duration, and dose; (c) sensitive to different components of exposure (e.g., alpha, beta, or gamma rays); (d) validated in similar conditions prior to their use, (e) quantitative and at least theoretically reproducible (f) complete, in that they covered all exposures for all involved people; and (g) accepted by all interested parties. As stated above, based on our own examination of the DNA dosimetry data, their consideration by others, we do not believe the data are appropriate for the individual-specific assignments necessary for the type of epidemiologic comparisons on which this report is based. We offer our justification of this decision in this section, along with a discussion of our consideration of alternative measures of dose, using subsets of the dosimetry data.

A Working Group of the Five Series Study Committee assessed the basis and quality of the data upon which dose assignments were made and concluded that they were not suitable for dose-response analyses in epidemiology (IOM 1995).

> The Working Group concluded that there has been a lack of consistency over time in NTPR dose estimation methods and, in particular, in the methods of assigning "high-sided" doses, that is, doses in which uncertainties are resolved in favor of assigning higher doses rather than lower doses. In some cases, because of the existing compensation program, procedures for assigning doses have been different for those who did and did not file a claim for a radiogenic cancer. Neither the dose assignment methods nor the database itself are thoroughly documented. In addition, uncertainties have not been estimated in a consistent manner and do not incorporate all potential sources of variability inherent in the dosimetry. (p. 2)

The conclusions also state, "Although there is anecdotal evidence that individual doses may have been greatly underestimated in individual cases, the overall tendency may have been to overestimate both external and internal doses."

The concurrence of both veterans with cancer having higher likelihood of individually reconstructed doses and reconstructed doses being more likely to be overestimated than others could introduce serious bias into the epidemiologic analysis of these data. However, the data may still be a useful indicator on a group basis in contrasting exposure surrogates in CROSSROADS. For their part, veterans have expressed concerns that the assigned doses are significantly lower than justified based upon their first-hand experiences at the test site.

Alternatives

Because the dose assignments are the subject of such hot debate, we looked for other indirect quantitative dose measures obtainable from the NTPR database. We hypothesized that either number of badges issued to an individual or total dose derived from badge data might be more reliable measures of individual exposure than the reconstructed total dose discussed above.

Based on DNA background material (DNA 1984), we hypothesized that participants most likely to be exposed to ionizing radiation would have been issued more badges than those believed less likely to be exposed. We looked, therefore, for relationships between the number of badges issued to an individual and both the total dose assigned to that individual and the dose assigned to that individual using badge data alone. Finding none, we rejected using number of badges as an exposure surrogate.

The badging in CROSSROADS was sparse—few people were badged and those who were did not wear their badges continuously during their exposure, according to participant and DNA accounts. Thus, an individual's cumulative dose from film badges may well give an incomplete picture of total dose in CROSSROADS. We examined the dosimetry data to determine if an individual's assigned dose was proportional to his badged dose, which would allow an assumption that badges were indicative of the total dose accrued by the individual. We found that individuals with very similar badged totals had widely disparate assigned doses due to differing dose reconstructions.

In summary, seeing no evidence that the film badge data provided a useful exposure surrogate, we chose not to use them.

PARTICIPANT VERSUS NONPARTICIPANT COHORTS AS AN EXPOSURE SURROGATE

Chapter 6 contains our discussion of the use of participation status as a proxy for exposure.

BOARDERS VERSUS NONBOARDING PARTICIPANTS VERSUS NONPARTICIPANTS AS EXPOSURE SURROGATES

One would expect individuals who boarded target ships after shot Able or Baker (or both) to be more highly exposed to radiation than others, since the ships were radiologically contaminated, in some cases very heavily. The boarders group does not correspond to a particular occupation; it consists of a variety of different enlisted ratings and officer ranks.

We define a boarder as someone who has a record of being on a target ship after one (or both) of the detonations or who has a unit designation of "RADSAFE" or "BOARDING TEAM." Ships assigned to CROSSROADS were categorized in DNA historical records as "target" or "support" ships. The former were literally the targets of the nuclear explosions. While all personnel were removed from target ships before the detonations, many reboarded those ships to monitor experiments, retrieve instruments, or decontaminate the vessel. Radiation safety officers were mostly medical and scientific personnel who carried radiation detection devices (e.g., Geiger counters) and were responsible for providing clearance or evacuation advice regarding other boarding party members. Boarding team personnel were so designated in their military assignment records.

This boarder variable has high face validity and makes what may be the best use of available data. The data, however, have not been validated regarding either accuracy of actual assignments or actual associations with ionizing radiation exposure. Furthermore, not all potential high-exposure groups are captured by the boarder variable. DNA narratives mention diving teams, for example, that may have been exposed but not recorded as such in assignment records (DNA 1984).

While the boarders represent a more exposed group of CROSSROADS participants, on balance the remaining participants constitute a less exposed group and the nonparticipants are an unexposed group. The distribution of individuals in occupation and grade categories and their status as boarders or nonboarders is reasonably balanced.

ENGINEERING & HULL VERSUS OTHER SPECIALTY STATUS AS AN EXPOSURE SURROGATE

An individual's military classification—by rank, rate, paygrade, or occupation—provides clues to his age, education, physical exposures, military salary, and postmilitary occupation (and concomitant exposures). While these classifications are relevant to this study as proxies for the confounding effects of socioeconomic characteristics (which we discussed in Chapter 3), in this section we consider their usefulness in developing proxies for an ionizing radiation exposure measure.

Military paygrades fell into three categories: enlisted (E1 to E7[18]), warrant officer (W1 to W4), and commissioned officer (O1 to O10). By the alphabetic letter we categorize—however grossly—something about the individual's position in the military hierarchy, while the number reflects, for one thing, time in service. Ranks provide service-specific nominal titles to the military-wide paygrades and provide descriptive information. Army examples of ranks are First Lieutenant (1LT, O2), Chief Warrant Officer (W2), and Staff Sergeant (E6). The Navy assigns ranks (for example, Captain, O6) to all officers, while a rating is assigned to all enlisted individuals. The rating combines information about a sailor's rank and occupational specialty (for example, Chief Electrician's Mate, E7, or Seaman Apprentice, E2). Navy enlisted ratings are unique in that they provide valuable information about typical duties. Similar information was unavailable to us for enlisted persons of other services or for officers of any service. We used the "Navy Career Path" (NAVPERS 1949) to reduce over a thousand variants of Navy ratings to 14 broad occupational specialty groups (Table 8-1).

TABLE 8-1. Broad Occupational Specialty Groupings of Navy Enlisted Ratings Developed from "Navy Career Paths" (1949)

Occupational Group	Major Job Fields (examples)
Administrative and Clerical	Communications Technician, Disbursing Clerk
Aviation	Aviation Machinist's Mate, Aviation Photographer's Mate
Construction	Surveyor, Steelworker
Deck	Boatswain's Mate, Radarman
Dental	Dental Technician
Electronics	Electronics Technician
Engineering & Hull	Boilerman, Machinist's Mate
Medical	Hospital Corpsman
Miscellaneous	Printer, Musician
Ordnance	Gunner's Mate, Mineman
Seaman	Seaman
Precision Equipment	Instrumentman, Opticalman
Steward	Steward, Cook
Unknown	No occupational information available

Each classification by itself has limitations for epidemiologic purposes. We therefore used the following criteria in our attempts to create a classification variable for our analyses:

[18]We have chosen for simplicity and clarity to use the modern designations for military paygrade—the terminology in use at the time of CROSSROADS was somewhat different.

- balanced cell sizes;
- provision of some information about potential exposure to ionizing radiation;
- provision of some control of unmeasured characteristics of individuals that could be related both to past, current, and future exposures and to health outcomes;
- efficient use of available information; avoidance of large unknown categories;
- a categorization that is both understandable to the reader and meaningful within a mortality analysis.

Prior nonmilitary research has shown that age, socioeconomic status, and occupation are all related to health outcomes. Naval Health Research Center reports associate specific occupations and grades with, for example, respiratory disease, mental disorders, accidents, and hospitalization rates (Gunderson 1976; Helmkamp and Colcord 1984; Helmkamp and Bone 1985a, 1985b). Available data do not include occupation or task-related information about officers. DNA materials (Appendix B) suggest that some job classifications may be associated with higher than normal radiation exposure potential at CROSSROADS. Because a major source of radiation at the CROSSROADS test site was contaminated seawater and because this seawater flowed through pipes in the Engineering & Hull spaces of the ships, one might expect individuals working in that environment to have been more highly exposed to radiation than other personnel. For that reason, DNA assigned higher doses to these individuals, based upon their Engineering & Hull rating. We therefore developed a seven-level variable (Table 8-2) that used information from occupational group and paygrade. We use this grouping in calculating standardized mortality ratios for Navy all-cause and all-malignancy mortality (Appendix C).

TABLE 8-2. General Rank/Rating and Occupational Specialty Categories for Navy Personnel

Engineering & Hull specialties, junior enlisted paygrades E1–E3
Engineering & Hull specialties, midlevel enlisted paygrades E4–E5
Engineering & Hull specialties, senior enlisted paygrades E6–E7
All other enlisted specialties, E1–E3
All other enlisted specialties, E4–E5
All other enlisted specialties, E6–E7
All officers, W1–W4 and O1–O10

There is great variability in occupation and activities within each of the above groups. Engineering & Hull occupations in the Navy are held by those individuals who were most likely to be found working below decks (Appendix

B). Included in this group are Boiler Tenders, Pipe Fitters, Machinists Mates, and similar enlisted ratings.

Other enlisted occupations range across Fire Control Technician, Steward, Journalist, Aviation Ordnanceman, and Accountant. Officers' responsibilities can include physical exposures in whatever area they command. Furthermore, paygrade provides a very imprecise and "noisy" measure of age and socioeconomic characteristics. For the enlisted men, we have incorporated three grade levels, junior (E1–E3), midlevel (E4–E5), and senior (E6–E7). There were insufficient numbers of officers to break them into grade subgroups while retaining statistical power. The combination of occupation and paygrade may also control for exposure potential determined in part by whether particularly "dirty" or "interesting" assignments were directed to junior or senior personnel.

RELATIONSHIPS OF SURROGATES WITH DNA DOSE DATA

Validating our surrogate measures is impossible without an accepted comparison standard. While holding to our critique of both measured (badged) and reconstructed doses to individuals, we recognize that those data may be useful for other than dose-response epidemiologic analyses with the individual as the unit of analysis.

We tabulated the surrogate measures of exposure described in this chapter—occupation, paygrade, boarder status, participant status—with the DNA dose estimates assigned to the personnel in those categories, thinking that general concordance would add support to our use of those surrogates. Note that this comparison was done in retrospect. Dose data were neither used nor considered in the conceptualization or development of the exposure surrogate variables. The validating comparisons were made after the decision was made to use the surrogates.

In retrospect, the DNA-assigned doses do confirm our exposure expectations in the surrogate groups we selected. Both the Engineering & Hull and the boarders[19] have higher assigned doses than those who are not in these categories. For the Engineering & Hull group, however, this is in some respects a self-fulfilling prophecy, since DNA increased their assigned dose estimates because they thought them to be at higher risk of exposure.

Our expectation of relatively high exposure in the RADSAFE and Able-only groups is reflected in both the badge and total assigned dose data. The total

---

[19]We separated boarders into three subcategories for this comparison: Able-only (individuals who boarded a target ship only in the period beginning after shot ABLE and ending with shot BAKER); Baker-only (individuals who boarded a target ship only in the period after shot BAKER); and both shots (individuals who boarded a target ship during both the Able-only and Baker-only periods defined above).

assigned dose data also validated our assumption of higher exposure in the Engineering & Hull, Baker-only, and both-shot groups. The badge data do not validate the last three groups, but their appropriateness as a validation tool is questionable because of the limitations of film badge dosimetry discussed earlier. Overall, we believe our selections of dose surrogate groups are consonant with the assigned total dose data and are not refuted by the badge data.

DECISIONS FOR THE ANALYSES IN THIS REPORT

Based on our considerations as described in the preceding sections, the committee and staff decided not to use dosimetry data in the analysis. This decision was not taken lightly. The amount of painstaking sifting through military records by DNA to develop the dose data was immense. So, too, is the information gained about a physical exposure that no one, until then, had been required to measure. The dose data, however, as previously described, do contain biases that could affect the study's results in ways that are not well defined. To prevent that, we made the decision not to use the individual-specific reconstructed or badged doses before looking at exposure-outcome correlations.

Our decisions on the establishment of dose surrogates were:

- Use participant vs. nonparticipant comparison.
- Use a consolidated boarder variable as one exposure surrogate.
- Use dosimetry data to provide an overall perspective regarding the amount of ionizing radiation exposure involved (see Appendix D).

9

Mortality Ascertainment

Whether we look at all-cause or disease-specific mortality, use standardized mortality ratios or proportional hazard modeling, adjust for a host of covariates or examine crude rates, the analysis hinges on having correctly ascertained mortality data. We need to know *who* died, *when*, and *of what cause or causes.*

Two pieces of information are essential: vital status (alive, dead, unknown) and cause of death (for those dead). We measure the data quality of these items on two scales: completeness (known, unknown) and correctness as determined by corroboration from other sources.

In this chapter we first describe this study's mortality ascertainment procedure, as planned given various constraints, and as adapted due to unforeseen and insurmountable obstacles. Appendix F consists of data illustrating the degree of success in achieving completeness and correctness. In closing this chapter, we discuss what effects that may have on the analysis and its interpretation.

PROCEDURE

Vital Status Ascertainment

Department of Veterans Affairs (VA) records are the core source of vital status information.[20] We begin with the Beneficiary Identification and Records Locator Subsystem (BIRLS), a computer file of VA transactions concerning benefits to individual veterans. Of particular interest to this study is the recording of death benefit requests. The BIRLS database fields include: name, claim number, claim folder location, Social Security Number, military service number(s), date of claim, claim folder location, and date of death.[21] BIRLS can be searched by automated routines using a standard protocol or by "hand," using whatever criteria the analyst seated at the terminal chooses.

Veterans were placed in one of three categories, depending on the success and findings of the BIRLS search.

- BIRLS record was found with reference to a death.
- BIRLS record was found with no reference to a death.
- BIRLS record was not found.

If the BIRLS record for an individual was not found, the next source searched was the Veterans Administration Master Index (VAMI). Now catalogued on microfilm, and replaced by the electronic BIRLS in the early 1970s, the VAMI had been maintained manually on 3 × 5 index cards, one for each veteran with a benefits claim. In addition to mortality information, VAMI is a source of other identifying information (e.g., different spelling of a name) that made subsequent BIRLS searches successful. VAMI searches must be done by hand.

Federal databases other than those maintained by the VA served as sources of vital status ascertainment. The Health Care Financing Administration (HCFA) of the Department of Health and Human Services (DHHS) searched its computerized database on Medicare enrollees and provided vital status on all reasonable to good potential matches, based on Social Security Number (SSN), date of birth, and name. As we discuss later in this section, HCFA information was used as one measure of the completeness of VA-based (BIRLS and VAMI) death information. All veterans not found in BIRLS plus a sample of veterans

---

[20]Although JAYCOR (for the Defense Nuclear Agency) constructed the participant cohort and MFUA staff constructed the comparison cohort, MFUA followed identical protocols for vital status follow-up of members of both cohorts, using the same data sources and search algorithms.

[21]Data fields available on BIRLS not relevant to this study are: insurance file and policy numbers, death in service, cause of death, power of attorney, dates of entry onto and release from active duty, branch of service, character of service, separation reason code, paygrade, and nonpay days.

found as Dead and found with no mention of death (presumed alive) were searched against the HCFA database for vital status.

The National Death Index (NDI), maintained for research purposes by the National Center for Health Statistics since its 1979 inception, assembles state death records. NDI searches its database by year for potential matches based on name, month and year of birth, and SSN. NDI provides the death certificate number—thereby confirming the fact of death—and the state possessing it.

After all available sources of vital status information were plumbed, the BIRLS-based categories were redefined into three categories for use in this study's analyses: Dead, Alive, and Lost to Follow-Up. If there was evidence of an individual's death, that veteran is coded "Dead"; if the veteran was found in BIRLS without reference to death, he was coded "Alive"; if a veteran was not found at all in BIRLS, he was coded "LTFU."

In the mortality analyses, we later collapse "Alive" and "LTFU" into a "Not Known Dead" category. (See Chapter 9.) Although this loses some detail about follow-up, it is the most accurate: a veteran is "Dead" or "Not Known to be Dead."

Cause and Date-of-Death Ascertainment

For individuals found in BIRLS and identified there as dead, BIRLS provided a date of death and VA claims folder location. MFUA requested a copy of the death certificate from the claims folder location and sent all death certificates to a certified nosologist, a specialist in classifying diseases. The nosologist wrote the four-digit ICD-9 codes for each cause of death listed on the death certificate, specifying one entry as the underlying cause of death and any others as associated causes of death.

Using the National Death Index (NDI)-provided death certificate number and state location, researchers can request, for another fee and a lengthy application assuring privacy protections, copies of the certificates from individual states. MFUA used NDI and state follow-up data as much as frugal efficiency would allow. In addition to their use in validating VA information, NDI findings also were used to fill gaps in VA data.

State vital records offices provided the death certificates of 908 veterans identified through NDI searches.

SUMMARY OF MORTALITY ASCERTAINMENT QUALITY AND ITS POTENTIAL EFFECTS ON VALID INTERPRETATION OF THE FINDINGS

VA databases were the primary sources of vital status information in this study. In order to confirm that these sources were appropriate, we checked them against two other sources: the Health Care Financing Administration (HCFA) and the National Death Index (NDI). In addition to this assurance that our mortality ascertainment through the VA sources was appropriate, we also checked on the consistency of our cause of death coding. These quality assurance procedures are documented in Appendix F. The results are discussed below.

Information on cause and date of identified deaths is available for 87.7 percent of the deaths included in this study's analyses (Appendix F, Table F-3). From our comparison of VA mortality data with that of NDI and HCFA, we found that our use of VA records to determine vital status is well justified. Use of other sources for variously selected samples did not yield substantially different results.

In addition, reliability of death coding according to the ICD-9 classification system, demonstrated by discrepancy rates of 4 percent for all-cause and 0.6 percent for leukemia (the primary hypothesized radiation-associated cancer), was good.

Discussion in Appendix F covers how this level of data quality was the best we could obtain for this study. Here, we discuss how the characteristics of our data, as well as the characteristics of mortality data in general, influence our interpretation of this study's findings.

Both HCFA and NDI validation samples indicate that MFUA's reliance on VA data sources yields only a small number of missed alleged deaths. HCFA and NDI, in turn, miss some VA-alleged deaths. None of the databases is a true standard. What may be more important to the interpretation of our findings is that the VA-missed (and, therefore, MFUA-missed) deaths are more prevalent among the participants than the controls. *If* participating in Operation CROSSROADS were associated with increased mortality, a differential in ascertainment between participants and controls could influence risk ratios if the differential were large enough relative to the expected numbers of deaths. The difference between 3.6 percent and 2.2 percent missed deaths (see Table F-8) is very small. For this study of 73,704 veterans with 22,896 deaths (as of 31 December 1992), we lose 344 deaths (1.5 percent x 31.1 percent x 73,704). If those missing deaths are evenly distributed across causes of death—and we have no evidence that they are not—the relative distribution of cause-specific mortality would not be affected and the risk ratio for all-cause mortality would diminish only slightly.

The less than 1 percent discrepancy in leukemia underlying cause-of-death coding is reassuring not only because of its small size, but also because it is likely to be dwarfed by other, unmeasured errors in cause-of-death coding. What is noted on a death certificate might be determined by—aside from the actual cause—competing diagnoses, inaccurate diagnoses, privacy concerns of the individual or the community, professional background of the signer, geographic practice patterns, and the decedent's health history and earlier access to medical care.

Cause of death as documented on a death certificate also varies over time: diagnoses come in and out of favor, and medical technology or knowledge may revise diagnostic criteria and categories. Over the course of the 50 years of mortality follow-up for this study, for example, terminology has been revised regarding lymphosarcoma and various dementias.

The basic comparisons in this study are based on all-cause mortality, which is generally a more accurate measure than cause-specific mortality. As for the specific cause of most interest in this study—leukemia—the reliability of that coding is excellent.

In summary, we found that our mortality ascertainment was very complete and well-balanced between participants and controls. If we were to take NDI and HCFA results as reliable indicators of missing deaths, the impact on our crude mortality would be either to increase participant mortality about 1.2 percent (using HCFA data) or to decrease it by 0.4 percent (using NDI data) relative to controls. Finally, the recoding of mortality causes suggests that any error induced from coding will be very small in comparison to other possible sources of error. We believe these mortality data may be used with confidence.

10

Characterization of the Cohorts and Analysis Plan

The overall goal of the analysis is to compare mortality among CROSSROADS participants with that among controls. In this chapter, we first describe the nature of the data on which that analysis rests and then describe the multivariate analysis plan itself. In an earlier chapter we presented data from the study, since some of the analytic strategies are influenced by our knowledge of our data's quality and idiosyncrasies. Data-based findings relating to the multivariate exposure-outcome relationships are presented in the following chapter (Chapter 11).

We have described in earlier chapters the detailed data collection plans and the practical adjustments that were necessary during their implementation. Refer to Chapter 5 for information on data sources. Chapters 6 and 7 describe *who* is in the analysis, while Chapters 8 and 9 discuss *what* data items are used and in what manner.

DATA DECISIONS TAKEN BEFORE ANALYSIS

Restricting Data Elements or Sample Definition

In the overall attempt to balance the validity, precision, understandability, and usefulness of the analyses in this report, we made the following decisions, based mostly on issues of data availability:

• Use the 1994 participant database provided by the Defense Nuclear Agency (DNA). (See Appendix E for a detailed description of procedures undertaken to validate the completeness of the participant roster.)

• Restrict analyses to Navy participants and controls (see Chapter 6).

• Do not include in participant cohort those individuals who came on duty in the CROSSROADS area of operations *after* the officially designated period of the operation (see Chapter 6).

• Exclude from the control cohort those also in the participant cohort (see Chapter 6).

• Include participants and controls who have other-than-CROSSROADS nuclear test participation (see Chapter 6).

• Use male mortality rates, since the control cohort is almost totally male (gender generally was not recorded on the research files for participants), when making comparisons to standard populations (e.g., the U.S. population for specific years). However, do not exclude female military personnel from the participant or control study cohorts.

• Do not use dosimetry; use exposure surrogate variables (see Chapter 8).

Data Cleaning and Variable Development

• Code vital status outcome as a dichotomy: "Known Dead" and "Not Known to be Dead." The latter included participants and controls known to be alive, having date of death after prearranged study cut-off (31 December 1992), and others for whom no death confirmation was obtained through the Department of Veterans Affairs (VA), who were presumed to be alive (see Chapter 9).

• For VA claims folders that did not contain a date of death from VA records or an acquired death certificate and that had been transferred from VA to a Federal Archives Record Center (FARC), use date of folder transfer to calculate an estimated date of death (see Chapter 9).

• Because military records used only two digits to designate year of birth, assign a century-of-birth prefix of "19" to years of birth 00 to 30 and the prefix "18" to years 31 to 99.

• Create a "boarder" variable to include participants assigned in the appropriate time period to one or more units known to be a target ship, a radiation safety unit, or a boarding team (see Chapter 8).

• Consolidate occupational specialty information into a two-level analysis variable (Engineering & Hull enlisted, other enlisted) to capture hypothesized exposure differences (see Chapter 8).

• Because of small numbers (paygrade and rank) or unavailable information (occupation), consider all officers as one category.

UNIVARIATE DESCRIPTIONS OF STUDY POPULATION

As we describe later in this chapter, we base our inferential comparisons on data adjusted for confounding influences on exposure-mortality relationships. Here, we present univariate (unadjusted) descriptive statistics on the variables used in later models. This information supports our belief that the Navy participant and control cohorts are similar in characteristics we can measure. Tables 10-1 through 10-3 show the numerical balance between participant and control cohorts for age, rank (or rating), and occupational specialty, respectively, for Navy personnel.

TABLE 10-1. Age-at-Shot Distribution of Navy Participants and Controls

		Participant Cohort		Control Cohort	
Age[a]	Years in Interval	No.	%	No.	%
≥ 16 and < 21	5	23,081	59.7	19,511	55.7
≥ 21 and < 26	5	9,504	24.6	9,365	26.7
≥ 26 and < 36	10	4,730	12.2	5,053	14.4
≥ 36 and < 46	10	1,134	2.9	962	2.7
≥ 46 and < 56	10	179	0.5	134	0.4
≥ 56 and < 66	10	11	0.0	2	0.0
≥ 66	2	2	0.0	1	0.0
Missing		27	0.1	8	0.0
Total[b]		38,668	100	35,036	100

[a] See Chapter 9 for discussion of the age variable.

[b] Mean age-at-shot for Navy participants is 22.06 years; for controls, 22.50.

TABLE 10-2. Distribution of Ranks and Ratings Among Navy Participants and Controls

	Participant Cohort		Control Cohort	
Paygrade*	No.	%	No.	%
E1 Junior Enlisted	12	0.0	10	0.0
E2 Junior Enlisted	10,624	27.5	9,773	27.9
E3 Junior Enlisted	7,321	18.9	6,616	18.9
E4 Midlevel Enlisted	5,377	13.9	4,881	13.9
E5 Midlevel Enlisted	4,917	12.7	4,225	12.1
E6 Senior Enlisted	4,316	11.2	3,752	10.7
E7 Senior Enlisted	2,718	7.0	2,330	6.7
W1 (Warrant) Officer	70	0.2	0	—
W2 (Warrant) Officer	425	1.1	477	1.4
W3 (Warrant) Officer	1	0.0	0	—
W4 (Warrant) Officer	1	0.0	0	—
O1 (Commissioned) Officer	934	2.4	1,186	3.4
O2 (Commissioned) Officer	719	1.9	786	2.2
O3 (Commissioned) Officer	526	1.4	491	1.4
O4 (Commissioned) Officer	338	0.9	259	0.7
O5 (Commissioned) Officer	194	0.5	167	0.5
O6 (Commissioned) Officer	157	0.4	74	0.2
O7 (Commissioned) Officer	0	—	0	—
O8 (Commissioned) Officer	10	0.0	1	0.0
O9 (Commissioned) Officer	4	0.0	0	—
O10 (Commissioned) Officer	2	0.0	0	—
Missing	2	0.0	8	0.0
Total	38,668	100	35,036	100

*See Chapter 8 for description of paygrade, rank, and rate.

TABLE 10-3. Distribution of Occupational Specialties Among Navy Participants and Controls

	Participant Cohort		Control Cohort	
Occupation*	No.	%	No.	%
Administrative and clerical	5,248	13.6	4,531	12.9
Aviation	920	2.4	519	1.5
Construction	322	0.8	285	0.8
Deck	2,444	6.3	2,204	6.3
Dental	1	0.0	0	—
Electronics	415	1.1	382	1.1
Engineering & Hull	9,399	24.3	8,756	25.0
Medical	639	1.7	582	1.7
Miscellaneous	459	1.2	401	1.1
Ordnance	1,455	3.8	1,343	3.8
Precision equipment	4	0.0	3	0.0
Seaman	13,776	35.6	12,481	35.6
Steward	213	0.6	101	0.3
Unknown	3,371	8.7	3,428	9.8
Missing	2	0.0	20	0.1
Total	38,668	100	35,036	100

*See Chapter 8 for description of Navy occupational specialties.

Participants are labeled as Nonboarding and Boarding and are present in the cohorts in numbers shown in Table 10-4.

TABLE 10-4. Distribution of Boarders in the Study Cohort

	Participant Cohort		Control Cohort	
Boarder*	No.	%	No.	%
Yes	8,996	23.3	0	0
No	29,672	76.7	35,036	100
Total (participants only)	38,668	100	35,036	100

*See Chapter 8 for discussion of boarder variable.

MISSING DATA

Imputation of Fact and Date of Death

Because we classified approximately 500 individuals as "Dead" solely because their VA claims folder had been transferred to a Federal Archive Records Center (FARC), we devised a test to determine whether such imputation of fact and date of death was justifiable. Looking at records with both noted dates of death and FARC transfer dates, we determined that there is a definite relationship between year of death and the date a claims folder is transferred to a FARC. We used the year-specific lag time for those known pairs to impute a lag time for date of death for those with only the FARC transfer date. For records transferred between 1956 and 1962, we adjusted the date to represent a death six years earlier. For 1963 to 1971 transfers, we used a three-year adjustment; for 1972 to 1985, two years; and for 1986 to 1995, one year.

Imputation of Date of Birth

For 1,448 otherwise complete Navy records, date of birth was missing. Since the proportional hazards and standardized mortality analyses we used require age information, we devised a date-of-birth imputation procedure. For individuals with known dates of birth in the participant and control cohorts, date of birth was associated with paygrade and military rating. We therefore used a missing data imputation technique (hot deck technique, Naus 1975) to assign a date of birth from a randomly selected member of the cohort. Records were first matched according to exact rating (e.g., Seaman) and paygrade (e.g., E2); those having no matching rated individual were assigned based on paygrade.

Summary

Table 10-5 describes the extent and distribution of missing data items by the important analysis categories of exposure and outcome.

TABLE 10-5. Number and Percent of Records With Missing Needed Data Item

		Participant Cohort		Control Cohort	
Characteristic	Denominator	No.	%	No.	%
Date of birth *without imputation*	All	873	2.25	610	1.74
Date of birth *with imputations*	All	27	0.07	8	0.02
Occupation	Enlisted	2	0.01	8	0.03
Paygrade	All	2	0.01	8	0.02
Date of death *without imputation*	Dead	401	3.32	166	1.54
Date of death *with imputations*	Dead	17	0.14	20	0.19
Cause of death	Dead	1,650	13.64	1,146	10.61

COMPLETENESS OF VITAL STATUS ASCERTAINMENT

Because recorded vital status is the main outcome in this study, differences in success in its ascertainment could distort the association we observe between exposure and that outcome. We discuss this in great detail in the preceding chapter (Chapter 9). In Tables 10-6 and 10-7 we present data on the follow-up of mortality status of participants and controls. Subjects are divided into those (1) known to have died and who have coded cause of death, (2) known to have died but with no cause of death available, (3) presumed alive (i.e., found on the Beneficiary Identification and Records Locator Subsystem [BIRLS] without a date of death or a FARC location), and (4) those not found on BIRLS, whom we consider lost to follow-up.

TABLE 10-6. Vital Status on Follow-Up

	Participants		Controls	
Vital Status on Follow-Up	No.	%	No.	%
Dead	12,093	31.3	10,806	30.8
Presumed alive	21,770	56.3	20,319	58.0
Lost to follow-up	4,805	12.4	3,911	11.2
Total	38,668	100	35,036	100

TABLE 10-7. Information Available on Deaths

	Participants		Controls	
Data Available on Deaths	No.	%	No.	%
Date and Cause	10,436	86.3	9,649	89.3
Date only	1,639	13.6	1,135	10.5
Cause only	7	0.1	10	0.1
Neither Cause nor Date	10	0.1	10	0.1
Blank	1	0.0	2	0.0
Total Dead	12,093	100	10,806	100

MORTALITY COMPARISONS

The overall goal of the analysis to is compare mortality among CROSSROADS participants with that among controls. Under the null hypothesis, which is usually defined as the absence of an association, there would be no differences in mortality rates between the participants and the controls. In particular, if participation at CROSSROADS had no effect, we would find no significant difference in overall mortality.

A secondary hypothesis arises from concerns that radiation exposure at CROSSROADS could be the cause of any effect that may be seen among participants relative to nonparticipating controls. Under this null hypothesis there would be no significant trend observed across boarding party participants (more exposure surrogate), non-boarding-party participants (less exposure surrogate), and nonparticipant controls (no exposure surrogate) in all-malignancy or leukemia mortality. Similarly, mortality experience in the

Engineering & Hull exposure group would be no different than that in the other enlisted group.

MULTIVARIATE ANALYSES

Cox Proportional Hazards Model

Using survival time since Operation CROSSROADS as the dependent variable, we use the proportional hazards model to estimate the risks associated with possible explanatory factors (e.g., participant status, boarder status, occupational specialty), including exposure, while mathematically adjusting for potential confounders (e.g., age, rank, rate, paygrade). This model, first formulated by Cox (1972), can take into account the varied lengths of follow-up and other time-dependent effects. We implemented the Cox analysis using the PHREG procedure in SAS (SAS Institute 1992). It is a semiparametric model that "measures the relative risk of death or disease in (infinitesimally) small time intervals under the assumption that the relative risk is constant over the follow-up period (Ingram and Makuc 1994)."

We used the Cox model with survival time as the response variable; vital status as the censoring variable;[22] and age, participant status, paygrade, Engineering & Hull status, and boarder status as explanatory variables. These covariate content areas were chosen before data collection; decisions regarding category divisions were informed by data availability and distributions. Variable definitions are found in Table 8.

Although the distributions of characteristics such as age and paygrade are similar for the participant and control cohorts, they are not identical, and thus we have adjusted for them in the analyses. This model estimates relative risk for one characteristic after removing the variation due to the distribution of other variables in the model. We present the output as relative rate ratios with 95 percent confidence intervals. All statistical tests are two-sided.

We examined the data for all-cause mortality, all-cancer mortality, leukemia mortality, and mortality from specific causes preselected because of concern or knowledge about radiogenicity. We tested a range of possible time-related interactions with exposure. To provide perspective, we also selected several broad categories of cause. The cause-of-death analysis categories are listed in Table 10-9 in decreasing categories of aggregation.

---

[22]For all-cause mortality, survival time is measured from 1 July 1946 to date of death; survivors are right censored at the end of the study (31 December 1992). For cause-specific mortality, survival time is measured from 1 July 1946 to date of death due to the specific cause; other deaths are right censored at time of death; survivors are right censored at the end of the study.

Table 10-8. Definitions of Analysis Variables

Variable Name	Definition*
Vital status	1 = Dead; 0 = Not Known Dead
Age at shot	Continuous variable calculated by date of shot minus date of birth
Survival time	Continuous variable calculated by date of death minus date of shot
Participant status	1 = Participant; 0 = Control
Boarder status	3-Level set of indicator variables representing boarding participants, nonboarding participants, and nonparticipant controls.
Paygrade	Paygrades summarized in four levels (junior enlisted, E1–E3; mid-level enlisted, E4–E5; senior enlisted, E6–E7; and Officers (commissioned and warrant, O1–O10 and W1–W4).
Occupation 1	3-Level set of indicator variables representing: Engineering & Hull, all other enlisted occupational specialties, and all officers.
Occupation 2	7-Level set of indicator variables combining information from 3-level Occupation 1 with 4-level paygrade categories.

*See Chapter 8 for a fuller description.

TABLE 10-9. ICD9 Mortality Codes Used as Case Definitions for Analyses

Case definition[a]	ICD9 mortality codes
All causes	0010–9999
All malignancies	1400–2021, 2024, 2027–2089, 2384, 2386, 2898
Buccal cancer	1400–1499
Digestive cancer	1500–1590, 1592–1599
Esophagal cancer	1500–1509
Stomach cancer	1510–1519
Large intestine cancer	1530–1539, 1590
Rectal cancer	1540–1542, 1544–1549
Liver cancer	1550–1551, 1553–1569
Pancreatic cancer	1570–1579
Respiratory cancer	1600–1639, 1642, 1643, 1648, 1649, 1650–1659
Lung cancer	1620–1629
Bone cancer	1700–1709
Skin cancer	1720-1739
Prostate cancer	1850–1859
Testicular cancer	1860–1876, 1878–1879
Bladder cancer	1880–1886, 1888–1889
Kidney cancer	1890–1899, 1887
Eye cancer	1900–1909
Brain and other CNS cancer	1910–1929
Thyroid cancer	1930–1939
All lymphopoietic cancer	2000–2021, 2024, 2027–2089, 2384, 2386, 2898
Lymphosarcoma and reticulosarcoma	2000–2009
Hodgkin's disease	2010–2019
Leukemia[b] and aleukemia	2040–2089, 2024, 2031
Other lymphatic tissue cancer	2020–2021, 2027–2030, 2032–2039, 2384, 2386, 2071, 2053, 1591
Multiple myeloma	2030, 2386
Benign neoplasms	2100–2376, 2378–2383, 2388–2399
Circulatory system disease	3900–4599
Respiratory disease	4600–5199
Digestive system disease	5200–5799
All external causes of death	8000–9989
All accidents	8000–9499
Motor vehicle accidents	8100–8299
Suicide	9500–9599
Infectious and parasitic diseases	001–139
Endocrine, nutritional, and metabolic diseases and immunity disorders	240–279

Diseases of the blood and blood-forming organs	280–289
Mental disorders	290–319
Diseases of the nervous system and sense organs	320–389
Diseases of the genitourinary system	580–629
Diseases of the skin and subcutaneous tissue	680–709
Diseases of the musculoskeletal system and connective tissue	710–739
Congenital anomalies	740–759
Symptoms, signs, and ill-defined conditions	780–799

[a]Case definitions chosen mostly from NCI updated mortality rates (NCI 1995); additional broad categories use ICD9 chapter headings as organizers (WHO 1995).
[b]For the proportional hazards analysis of leukemia, we excluded chronic lymphoid leukemia because it has not been identified as radiogenic. The software package for SMR calculations, however, includes CLL (Preston et al. 1993).

Standardized Mortality Ratios

For comparison with other atomic veteran studies (Darby 1988, 1993; NRC 1985) we calculated standardized mortality ratios (SMRs) for all-cause mortality, all malignancies, and leukemias for the Navy, Marine, and Army cohorts. To control for age and social factors in all-cause and all-malignancy categories, we calculated separate SMRs by the seven-level "Occupation 2" variable described in Table 8-2, Chapter 8. For leukemias, where there were few cases, we collapsed the seven levels over rank and rating. We expected that both participants and controls would exhibit a "healthy soldier effect." The details of this secondary analysis are presented in Appendix C.

An oft-raised and truly considerable drawback to SMR use in studies of occupational-type exposures is the healthy worker—or soldier (sailor)—effect described in Chapter 3. In fact, an earlier National Research Council mortality study of atmospheric nuclear tests and mortality (Robinette et al. 1985) was criticized for using SMRs as its sole risk comparison. The study we report here was designed to include a military reference cohort to provide a finer comparison. The SMR comparison to the U.S. white male population[23] of the period under study adds, as mentioned above, a perspective that is useful as long as one keeps its limitations in mind.

[23]Navy personnel in 1946 were predominantly white; we have no individual data on race.

ANALYSIS OF ARMY (INCLUDING ARMY AIR CORPS) AND MARINE DATA

The Navy constituted 91 percent of the CROSSROADS cohort, has occupational specialty information available on its enlisted component, has the largest availability of identification data (availability of date of birth in participants, 97.8 percent, and controls, 98.3 percent) and the most complete cause-of-death information (89.3 percent controls/86.3 percent participants). For that reason we chose to do our primary analysis on the Navy data.

For the Army, which was 7.8 percent of the CROSSROADS cohort, fully 20.4 percent of the dates of birth in the participants were missing and had to be imputed (as compared to 1.8 percent for controls). In addition, the availability of causes of death was lower for Army than for Navy personnel (87.9 percent for participants, 85.9 percent for controls). The quality for the Marines was comparable to that of the Navy, but the Marines constitute a comparatively small number of individuals (557 participants), making detailed analysis of the group impossible from a statistical point of view. Because the Marines do not have any specialty information available for their enlisted ranks, we were reluctant to mix them in with the Navy data.

As a result of these factors, we chose to:

- analyze the Army and the Marine data for differences in all-cause, all-cancer, and leukemia mortality using the proportional hazards model developed for the Navy without the occupational specialty variables, and
- compute SMRs on the Army and Marines only for all-cause, all-cancer, and leukemia mortality.

We do these analyses with some hesitation, given the limitations in the Army data and the small number of Marines, and we present the results solely for completeness. The conclusions of the study are based entirely upon our findings among the Navy personnel.

NOT THE SUBJECT OF ANALYSIS IN THIS REPORT

As we have stated before, this study was designed and funded subject to several unavoidable constraints, among which are: dosimetry is incomplete; military records do not keep the type of data often required for epidemiologic investigation, and those data items that are kept are not always complete; the U.S. does not have a centralized national vital statistics database for individuals that spans the time period 1946 until now; cause-of-death data have known limitations; Operation CROSSROADS was only one event in a lifetime of physical and psychological events for the participants; and few women were assigned to units included in participant and control cohorts.

For these reasons, this report neither explores nor addresses all the interesting facets of possible exposure-outcome associations. It can, therefore, neither reassure nor vindicate those who feel strongly about the nature of many of those associations. Areas of inquiry into which we have not delved in this study but for which we could imagine a study design include:

- exposure-outcome analyses based on exact dosimetry estimates calculated for a subset of the overall study population;
- fuller examination of cause of death, looking beyond the underlying cause to all associated or contributory causes listed on the death certificate; and
- detailed analysis of the participants who served in the Marines and Army (including the Army Air Corps) in CROSSROADS and their controls.

Unfortunately, the following group of topics may never be well studied in this observational cohort due to reasons including very small numbers; the nonexistence of necessary exposure information; and the unfeasibility, if not impossibility, of tracking health outcomes other than death:

- unique aspects, if any, of the exposure-outcome relationship in women;
- possible effects of participation or other measures of exposure on outcomes other than mortality, looking at morbidity rates for the diseases considered in the mortality study (e.g., skin cancer) and for other diseases and conditions believed to be radiogenic (e.g., cataracts);
- adverse reproductive outcomes;[24]
- more finely defined categories of military occupation, for officers and non-Navy enlisted personnel for whom no occupation data is available; and
- the interrelationships of other, non-CROSSROADS, risk factors accruing before, during, and after the Operation CROSSROADS activities, including an overlapping array of exposures that could be chemical and physical (occupational, environmental, behavioral); socioeconomic (education, income, occupation); geographic; and medical (comorbidities). Not the least of these is the possibility that many of the participants, as a result of their special radiological training for Operation CROSSROADS, may have gone on to careers associated with radiation.

---

[24]Feasibility is discussed in Institute of Medicine, Medical Follow-up Agency. *Adverse Reproductive Outcomes in Families of Atomic Veterans: The Feasibility of Epidemiologic Studies.* Washington, D.C.: National Academy Press, 1995.

11

Findings and Discussion

ORGANIZATION

The core question of this study concerns whether exposure to ionizing radiation at Operation CROSSROADS increased mortality. For reasons described earlier (and discussed again later) in this report, we approached this question from three directions. First, hypothesis A compares all participants to all nonparticipant controls to answer whether being a participant at CROSSROADS is associated with mortality. To hone in on whether ionizing radiation might be a causal factor in the relative mortality experiences of participants and controls, we then divide participants into boarding and nonboarding groups to test the hypothesized ionizing radiation exposure gradient as hypothesis B. Finally, based on the Defense Nuclear Agency (DNA) assertion that Navy personnel assigned to Engineering & Hull occupational specialties may have been exposed to radiation via pipes carrying contaminated water (Appendix B), we also examine, as hypothesis C, the association of Engineering & Hull status (as a radiation exposure measurement surrogate) with mortality.

We present the findings in this section from these three directions of inquiry:

- Model A. BASIC

To test effect of participant status on mortality. Independent variables are:

participant status (1 = yes; 0 = no)
age on 1 July 1946 (continuous)
paygrade categories:
junior enlisted (baseline)
mid-level enlisted
senior enlisted
officer

- Model B. BOARDER GRADIENT

To test effect of boarding status (see Chapter 10) as a stronger radiation exposure surrogate than participant status alone, the model substitutes for the participant status variable two indicator variables creating a hypothesized gradient of radiation exposure:

nonparticipant control (baseline)
nonboarding participant (level 1 exposure)
boarding participant (level 2 exposure)

- Model C. ENGINEERING & HULL

To test effect of the Engineering & Hull occupational category as a radiation exposure surrogate. Includes parameters of the basic model (A), less participant status—participants and controls are tested separately. A variable for Engineering & Hull status is added:

Engineering & Hull status (1 = yes, 0 = no)

Major mortality endpoints are: (1) all-cause, (2) all-malignancies, and (3) leukemias and aleukemias, excluding chronic lymphoid leukemia (CLL). Other descriptive mortality rates are presented by level of aggregation within cause of death (e.g., selected major categories, selected causes within selected major categories, etc.).

In developing the models displayed, we considered alternative modeling of variables, the role of other available data elements, and potential interactions among exposures and personnel characteristics. The tests that revealed no information are not displayed in these tables but are described later in this section.

In Tables 11-1 through 11-8 we display rate ratios calculated from estimated proportional hazards parameters for the first two models (A, participation effects, and B, boarding effects), using survival time as the response variable, censored as necessary at the end of the study follow-up period (31 December 1992). Results of Model C (Engineering & Hull effects) are presented separately in Tables 11-9. Because occupational specialty, of which the Engineering & Hull designation is one, is available only for enlisted personnel, we exclude officers from the analysis in Model C.

FINDINGS: DISPLAYED IN TABLES

Tables 11-1 through 11-8 display the rate ratios computed from the Cox proportional hazards model comparing participants with nonparticipants. As noted above, Model A considers all participants as an exposed group. Model B attempts to measure a hypothesized exposure gradient, with boarding participants as the most likely to be exposed to radiation hazard, nonboarding participants as less likely to be so exposed, and nonparticipants (controls) as unexposed. The display includes all tested causes of death.

Model C generated rate ratios in Table 11-9 associated with Engineering & Hull status for participants and controls separately, when included in a model along with age and paygrade.

TABLE 11-1. Rate Ratios of Major Mortality Endpoints for Exposed to Not-Exposed Personnel

		A: Basic[a]	B: Boarder Gradient[a]	
Case Definition[b]	No. of Deaths	All Participants[c]	Nonboarding Participants[d]	Boarding Participants[e]
All causes[f,g]	22,847[h]	**1.046 (1.020–1.074)**[i]	**1.043 (1.015–1.073)**	**1.057 (1.014–1.102)**
All malignancies[f,g]	5,647	1.014 (0.962–1.068)	1.010 (0.955–1.068)	1.026 (0.943–1.116)
Leukemia +aleukemia[f]	163	1.020 (0.750–1.387)	1.024 (0.737–1.422)	1.007 (0.610–1.663)

Notes for Tables 11-1 through 11-8:

[a]Analyses based on 73,704 Navy participants and controls.
[b]Table 10-9 in Chapter 10 provides complete category names and ICD9 codes.
[c]All participants relative to all controls, adjusting for age and paygrade.
[d]Non-boarding participants relative to all controls, adjusting for age and paygrade.
[e]Boarding participants relative to all controls, adjusting for age and paygrade.
[f]An *a priori* hypothesis based on ionizing radiation literature.
[g]Subsets in later table.
[h]Records of 12 deaths for which a necessary variable was missing or out of range were dropped from this analysis.
[i]Rate ratios from SAS PHREG procedure for proportional hazard ratios with 95 percent confidence intervals; boldface if confidence interval does not contain 1.00 (statistically significant at .05 level)

TABLE 11-2. Mortality Rate Ratios from Six Selected Major Cause-of-Death Categories (Subset of Table 11-1)

		A: Basic	B: Boarder Gradient	
Case Definition	No. of Deaths	All Participants	Nonboarding Participants	Boarding Participants
Benign neoplasm	63	0.969 (0.591–1.590)	1.065 (0.635–1.785)	0.654 (0.254–1.683)
Circulatory disease	8,447	1.011 (0.968–1.055)	1.012 (0.967–1.059)	1.008 (0.940–1.080)
Digestive disease	1,005	1.089 (0.962–1.234)	1.088 (0.953–1.242)	1.094 (0.898–1.332)
External cause	2,519	1.025 (0.948–1.109)	1.009 (0.927–1.097)	1.079 (0.955–1.219)
Malignant neoplasm[f,g]	5,647	1.014 (0.962–1.068)	1.010 (0.955–1.068)	1.026 (0.943–1.116)
Respiratory disease	1,174	1.070 (0.954–1.201)	1.053 (0.931–1.191)	1.129 (0.943–1.352)

TABLE 11-3. Mortality Rate Ratios from Remaining Major Cause-of-Death Categories (Subset of Table 11-1)

		A: Basic	B: Boarder Gradient	
Case Definition	No. of Deaths	All Participants	Nonboarding Participants	Boarding Participants
Blood-forming	37	1.221 (0.637–2.340)	1.353 (0.690–2.653)	0.769 (0.224–2.642)
Congenital	24	0.910 (0.408–2.028)	0.778 (0.317–1.905)	1.377 (0.444–4.276)
Endocrine	317	1.155 (0.925–1.441)	1.248 (0.990–1.574)	0.848 (0.572–1.258)
Genitourinary	181	0.876 (0.654–1.172)	0.899 (0.659–1.228)	0.795 (0.480–1.317)
Ill-defined	431	**0.769 (0.636–0.930)**	**0.769 (0.626–0.944)**	0.770 (0.559–1.059)
Infectious	200	1.045 (0.792–1.380)	0.984 (0.728–1.330)	1.254 (0.827–1.903)
Mental	152	0.963 (0.701–1.324)	0.927 (0.657–1.309)	1.084 (0.661–1.775)
Musculoskeletal	0	—	—	—
Nervous	236	1.107 (0.856–1.430)	1.105 (0.841–1.452)	1.112 (0.738–1.675)
Skin	16	1.209 (0.450–3.247)	1.223 (0.429–3.488)	1.162 (0.241–5.597)

TABLE 11-4. Mortality Rate Ratios from Selected Cancer Sites within All Malignancies (Table 11-2)

		A: Basic	B: Boarder Gradient	
Case Definition	No. of Deaths	All Participants	Nonboarding Participants	Boarding Participants
Bladder	90	0.964 (0.638–1.458)	0.868 (0.550–1.369)	1.292 (0.708–2.358)
Bone	18	0.912 (0.362–2.299)	0.922 (0.343–2.479)	0.876 (0.189–4.060)
Brain/CNS	164	0.827 (0.609–1.125)	0.771 (0.550–1.081)	1.013 (0.634–1.618)
Buccal	159	0.983 (0.720–1.342)	1.040 (0.749–1.443)	0.792 (0.455–1.377)
Digestive[g]	1,247	1.021 (0.913–1.141)	1.039 (0.923–1.170)	0.959 (0.798–1.153)
Eye	137	1.100 (0.786–1.540)	1.096 (0.766–1.569)	1.112 (0.651–1.901)
Kidney	0	—	—	—
Lymphopoietic[g]	480	0.975 (0.815–1.166)	0.909 (0.747–1.105)	1.198 (0.915–1.567)
Prostate	292	**0.767 (0.609–0.966)**	0.796 (0.623–1.018)	0.668 (0.441–1.011)
Respiratory[g]	2,354	1.036 (0.956–1.124)	1.039 (0.953–1.133)	1.028 (0.902–1.171)
Skin	128	0.817 (0.577–1.157)	0.870 (0.602–1.257)	0.643 (0.340–1.217)
Testicular	24	0.763 (0.341–1.705)	0.814 (0.347–1.909)	0.593 (0.134–2.631)
Thyroid	9	3.479 (0.720–16.81)	3.248 (0.628–16.80)	4.235 (0.593–30.24)

TABLE 11-5. Mortality Rate Ratios for Selected Cancer Sites within Digestive, Respiratory, and Lymphopoietic Cancers (Subset of Table 11-4)

Case Definition	No. of Deaths	A: Basic All Participants	B: Boarder Gradient Nonboarding Participants	 Boarding Participants
Esophagus	177	1.165 (0.866–1.568)	1.227 (0.898–1.677)	0.962 (0.582–1.588)
Hodgkin's Disease	45	0.748 (0.415–1.347)	0.536 (0.264–1.090)	1.444 (0.673–3.097)
Large intestine	422	0.931 (0.769–1.127)	0.946 (0.771–1.160)	0.883 (0.642–1.215)
Leukia+aleuk.[f]	163	1.020 (0.750–1.387)	1.024 (0.737–1.422)	1.007 (0.610–1.663)
Liver	55	1.492 (0.866–2.572)	1.533 (0.866–2.712)	1.355 (0.576–3.188)
Lung	2,252	1.048 (0.965–1.139)	1.056 (0.966–1.153)	1.024 (0.895–1.170)
Lymphos.+Reticul.	71	0.998 (0.627–1.591)	0.767 (0.449–1.313)	1.787 (0.973–3.283)
Other lymphatic[g]	169	1.021 (0.755–1.381)	0.998 (0.721–1.380)	1.100 (0.686–1.763)
Pancreas	240	1.114 (0.864–1.436)	1.122 (0.856–1.470)	1.085 (0.720–1.635)
Rectum	88	0.844 (0.556–1.283)	0.781 (0.493–1.237)	1.060 (0.561–2.002)
Stomach	194	1.038 (0.783–1.376)	1.139 (0.849–1.529)	0.703 (0.413–1.196)

TABLE 11-6. Mortality Rate Ratio for Selected Subset of Other Lymphatic Tissue (Subset of Table 11-5)

Case Definition	No. of Deaths	A: Basic All Participants	B: Boarder Gradient Nonboarding Participants	 Boarding Participants
Multiple myeloma	65	0.893 (0.549–1.453)	0.978 (0.588–1.628)	0.608 (0.237–1.559)

TABLE 11-7. Mortality Rate Ratios for Subset of External Causes (Subset of Table 11-2)

		A: Basic	B: Boarder Gradient	
Case Definition	No. of Deaths	All Participants	Nonboarding Participants	Boarding Participants
All accidents[g]	1,600	0.975 (0.884–1.076)	0.962 (0.865–1.069)	1.019 (0.873–1.190)
All suicides	525	1.030 (0.867–1.223)	0.958 (0.795–1.156)	1.262 (0.980–1.624)

TABLE 11-8. Mortality Rate Ratio for Subset of All Accidents (Subset of Table 11-7)

		A: Basic	B: Boarder Gradient	
Case Definition	No. of Deaths	All Participants	Nonboarding Participants	Boarding Participants
Motor vehicle accidents	778	0.929 (0.807–1.070)	0.922 (0.792–1.073)	0.953 (0.762–1.192)

TABLE 11-9. Rate Ratios for All-Cause Mortality of Engineering & Hull to Non-Engineering & Hull Groups by Status as Participants or Controls

Case Definition[b]	No. of Deaths	Engineering & Hull PARTICIPANTS[a,j]	No. of Deaths	Engineering & Hull CONTROLS[a,j]
All causes[f]	10,811	0.995 (0.953–1.038)[h]	9,562	0.979 (0.936–1.024)
All malignancies[f]	2,620	1.051 (0.965–1.144)	2,403	1.032 (0.945–1.127)
Leukemia+aleukemia[f]	74	1.515 (0.940–2.442)	69	1.292 (0.786–2.125)

Notes for Table 11-9:

[a]Analyses based on 66,872 Navy enlisted personnel, participants and controls.

[b]Table 10-9, Chapter 10 provides complete category names and ICD9 codes.

[j]Enlisted personnel in Engineering & Hull specialties relative to enlisted personnel in other occupational specialties, adjusted for age and paygrade only.

[f]An *a priori* hypothesis based on ionizing radiation literature.

NARRATIVE SUMMARY OF FINDINGS

Participant Status

All-Cause Mortality (Table 11-1)

The participants in CROSSROADS had a 4.6 percent higher mortality in comparison to the nonparticipants (p = .0006), relative risk (RR) = 1.046, 95% confidence interval, 1.020–1.074. Age at CROSSROADS and paygrade confirmed known mortality risks: increasing age and decreasing paygrade are associated with increasing mortality.

Mortality from All Malignancies (Table 11-2)

Participants experienced a slightly higher (1.4 percent) mortality from malignant neoplasms, RR = 1.014 (0.962–1.068), but this could be due to chance (p = 0.2579).

Mortality from Leukemia (including leukemias and aleukemias, excluding CLL) (Table 11-5)

Participant mortality was 2 percent higher than for the comparable controls RR = 1.020 (0.750–1.387). However, these results could again have been due to chance (p = 0.8992).

Mortality from Other Selected Causes (Tables 11-2 through 11-8)

The excess in all causes of mortality did not appear to be concentrated in any one of the subcategories of mortality studied, and none of the subcategory differences was statistically significant. We note that both nonmalignant respiratory disease and respiratory cancer showed elevated but not significant relative risks. In addition, ill-defined causes and prostate cancer showed significantly decreased mortality risks of 0.769 (0.636–0.930), p = 0.0067, and 0.767 (0.609–0.966), p = 0.0243, respectively, but this could be a result of chance, given the large numbers of comparisons made.

Boarder Status/Hypothesized Exposure Gradient

All-Cause Mortality (Table 11-1)

Both the nonboarders and boarders had significantly elevated mortality relative to controls (relative risks with 95% confidence intervals of 1.043 [1.015–1.073], p = 0.0028 and 1.057 [1.014–1.102], p = 0.0093, respectively). However, the risk to boarding participants is not significantly different from nonboarding participants (tested formally[25] and most easily seen by the overlapping confidence intervals), and these differences may be due to chance.

Mortality from All Malignancies (Table 11-2)

Although both nonboarders and boarders had slightly elevated mortality due to all malignancies relative to controls (relative risks of 1.010 [0.955–1.068], p = 0.7284 and 1.026 [0.943–1.116], p = 0.5502, respectively), these differences were not significant.

Mortality from Leukemia (Table 11-5)

Again, both nonboarders and boarders had slightly increased leukemia mortality (relative risks of 1.024 [0.737–1.422], p = 0.8879 and 1.007 [0.610–1.663], p = 0.9778, respectively) relative to controls, but these differences were not statistically significant and could be due to chance.

Other Selected Causes of Death (Tables 11- 2 through 11- 8)

Mortality risk from ill-defined disease was significantly lower in the nonboarding participants than in the controls (relative risk of 0.769 [0.626–0.944], p = 0.0119). Risks of mortality from other diseases considered were not statistically significant, and the decrease in ill-defined disease could be due to chance, given the large number of comparisons made.

[25]We also considered models (not displayed in this report) that included a boarder status indicator variable along with a participant status indicator variable. In these models, where the nonboarders included nonboarding participants as well as controls, the parameter estimates for boarder status were not significant.

Engineering & Hull Status/Hypothesized Exposure Surrogate

All-Cause Mortality (Table 11- 9)

Enlisted participants whose occupational specialty was Engineering & Hull experienced lower all-cause mortality than participants in other occupational specialties—relative risk with 95 percent confidence intervals of 0.995 (0.953–1.038), but the difference was not significant (p = .8059). A similar pattern was seen within the controls (relative risk 0.979 [.0936–1.024], p = 0.3542).

Mortality from All Malignancies (Table 11-9)

Engineering & Hull enlisted participants experienced 5.1 percent higher mortality than those in other occupational specialties (relative risk of 1.051 [0.965–1.144]), although the difference could be attributable to chance (p = 0.2529). As with all-cause mortality, the increase in the controls was slightly less, but again statistically not significant (relative risk, 1.032 [0.945–1.127], p = 0.4845).

Mortality from Leukemia (Table 11-9)

As seen in the all-cause and all-malignancies categories above, the Engineering & Hull participants showed increased mortality (relative risk 1.515 [0.940–2.442]), but the difference was not statistically significant (p = 0.0879). Mortality from leukemia in the controls was also elevated, but not as much (relative risk 1.292 [0.786–2.125], p = 0.3130). Once again, the differences are not statistically significant and could be due to chance.

FINDINGS FOR MARINES AND ARMY (INCLUDING ARMY AIR CORPS) PERSONNEL

Navy personnel constitute 91 percent of CROSSROADS participants. For that and other reasons discussed in Chapter 10, our report focuses on those personnel. Here, we present parallel tables with data from the Marines (Table 11-10) and the Army (including Army Air Corps, Table 11-11). Only Navy personnel had boarder or Engineering & Hull status assigned; we therefore consider only the basic participant versus control comparison for the other services.

TABLE 11-10. Mortality Rate Ratios of Participants Relative to Controls (Marines, n = 1,137)

Case Definition	No. of Deaths	All Participants
All causes	346	1.059 (0.857–1.308)
All malignancies	81	**1.711 (1.092–2.680)**
Leukemias	4	0.358 (0.037–3.489)

The increased risk of death from malignant neoplasms should be explored in a larger cohort to confirm this apparent increase. The standardized mortality ratios for all-malignancies were 0.5858 (0.3796–0.7921) for Marine controls and 0.9524 (0.6801–1.225) for the participants. For the complete Navy cohort they were: for controls, 0.8156 (0.7846–0.8465), and for participants, 0.8196 (0.7895–0.8497). The Marine controls appeared significantly healthier than either the Navy participants or the Navy controls. The apparent increase in all-malignancy mortality may be a deficit in the control population; the small size of the Marine cohort may exaggerate instabilities in the data. We cannot dismiss the possibility that this is a chance finding among the many comparisons made in this analysis. More definitive information will be available at the conclusion of the ongoing Five Series Study, which has a Marine cohort 10 times the size of the one in CROSSROADS.

TABLE 11-11. Mortality Rate Ratios of Participants Relative to Controls (Army, including Army Air Corps, n = 6,482)

Case Definition	No. of Deaths	All Participants
All causes	2,454	**0.754 (0.694–0.818)**
All malignancies	542	**0.777 (0.652–0.926)**
Leukemias	15	0.775 (0.270–2.219)

Deficits in both all-cause mortality and all-malignancy mortality are statistically significant. Preliminary explorations of Army data suggest problems with the control cohorts assembled. Although we based control selection on the rank distribution of the participant cohort, we did not have the education information available that would permit a finer selection. Because Army officers were selected for Operation CROSSROADS to perform high-level technical and scientific tasks, they were probably more highly educated than a random set of Army officers—a characteristic associated in other studies with better health outcomes. Thus, there could well be a mismatch in education level between Army participants and controls. A comparison of the two groups might yield an apparent and erroneous impression that CROSSROADS participation was associated with better health, a "protective" effect. While this may be true of Navy officers also, the effect would be larger in the Army, where 28.3 percent of the cohort were officers, compared to the 8.7 percent in the Navy.

In addition to these problems, the Army at the time of CROSSROADS included the Army Air Corps. There is some ambiguity in the rank structure between the mid-level and senior-level Army enlisted personnel. As a result there is an imbalance in these ranks between the control and participant cohorts for a relatively small number of men. Finally, we are still missing dates of birth for approximately 21 percent of the Army participants. Because we have imputed missing dates from randomly selected cohort members with the same rank and paygrade, misclassifications in rank assignments could influence the age variable. For all these reasons, we are not well assured that the findings for the Army subcohort of this study are valid. We present them here for completeness.

DISCUSSION

Boarders

Navy personnel who, according to records, boarded target ships during the CROSSROADS period following either or both detonations are the most clearly identifiable group of participants exposed to ionizing radiation on contaminated target ships. Hence, as we discussed in Chapter 8, those 8,996 participants represent a more highly exposed surrogate group.

If radiation following the atmospheric nuclear tests at CROSSROADS influenced the subsequent mortality of participants, we would expect its influence to be most concentrated among the boarders. A dose-response relationship could be hypothesized with controls at no dose, nonboarding participants at some dose, and boarding participants at a higher dose. (It also is possible that "boarding" could have entailed other, unidentified risks that affected later mortality. We are not aware of such factors, nor have others proposed examples.) Such a dose-response relationship is not observed in these data. A clear indication of a radiation effect would be a gradient with the some-dose group (participant nonboarders) having significantly higher risk than the no-dose group (controls) and the higher-dose group (participant boarders) having significantly higher risk than the some-dose group. This lack of association could indicate: (1) radiation from CROSSROADS detonations did not affect mortality, (2) the precision in assigning boarder status was inadequate to ensure accurate exposure classification, making a finding of no association uninformative, or (3) risks were present but were too small to be detected in a cohort of this size.

Boarders did, however, show increased mortality risk estimates relative to the control cohort—though not attaining statistical significance—in the ICD9 categories for Lymphosarcoma and Reticulosarcoma (RR = 1.787 [0.973–3.283]) and Hodgkin's Disease (RR = 1.444 [0.673–3.097]), both within the broader category of lymphopoietic cancers. When comparing the approximately 9,000 boarders to the *controls and the nonboarding participants* combined,[26] the rate ratios increase to 2.447 for lymphosarcoma and reticulosarcoma and 2.971 for Hodgkin's Disease, both reaching statistical significance. This difference in risk estimates reflects the inclusion in the comparison group of the much lower risk nonboarding participants. Possible explanations—none of which can be tested within the available data—are: (1) radiation is associated with increased risk of lymphosarcoma and reticulosarcoma and Hodgkin's Disease; (2) some unidentified nonradiation exposure associated with boarder status is also associated with increased mortality risk for those cancers; or (3) the boarder-cancer association is observed by chance, quite possible in this study with the large numbers of comparisons considered.

While earlier medical literature on radiation and cancer posed a possible relationship for these types of cancers (Upton 1982), a recent compilation of radiation effects specifically states that these types of cancer are not likely to be radiogenic (NRC 1990). Pierce (1996) found no significant dose effect for lymphoma in the atomic bomb survivor cohort. However, clinicians and researchers have identified problems with these diagnostic categories and created new disease classification schemes by which to describe types of lymphomas. These newer classifications replacing lymphosarcoma and reticulosarcoma use both histologic and morphologic criteria. We cannot determine what revised diagnoses might be coded from the observed lymphoma deaths in our dataset using the newer, more descriptive terminology. It is possible that these cancers would then fit into categories considered radiogenic; we may have identified a hitherto undescribed association or, as mentioned earlier, this may be a chance finding.

Engineering & Hull

In its attempt to assign doses to CROSSROADS participants, DNA considered personnel assigned to Engineering & Hull occupations as a potential high exposure group (see Chapter 8 and Appendix D for more detail). We tested whether that dichotomy was associated with mortality among enlisted personnel (these assignment data were not available for officers).

Our analyses were designed to test whether Engineering & Hull personnel had higher mortality, after mathematically adjusting for paygrade and age. There were no statistically significant elevations of mortality from all causes, malignancies, or leukemias in the Engineering & Hull group of participants compared to the non-Engineering & Hull group. More important, comparisons

[26]In the model comparing the 9,000 boarders to the controls and nonboarding participants combined, lymphosarcoma and reticulosarcoma and Hodgkin's Disease were the only 2 of 44 causes of death tested to reach statistical significance at the 0.05 level.

within the controls also yielded similar and nonsignificant results. These findings do not support a hypothesis that Engineering & Hull personnel experienced higher mortality due to radiation exposure at CROSSROADS. This lack of association could indicate: (1) radiation from CROSSROADS detonations did not affect mortality, (2) Engineering & Hull status was an inadequate exposure surrogate for radiation dose, making a finding of no association uninformative, or (3) risks were present but were too small to be detected in a cohort of this size.

Discussion of Other Findings

The tables provided earlier in this section display some risk estimates that, while not achieving statistical significance, may be useful topics for discussion and further exploration. We display in Table 11-12 the risk estimates that indicate at least a 40 percent excess (RR $\geq$ 1.4) or a 40 percent deficit (RR $\leq$ 0.6) risk related to CROSSROADS participation or boarder status. Most of these are based on small numbers of deaths and are not statistically significant. It should be noted that when many comparisons are made, a few will show a large rate ratio by chance alone.

By mathematical definition, a random 5 percent of numerous comparisons might show statistical significance at the 0.05 level regardless of biological causation, with about half of the point estimates being raised and the other half lowered. Similarly, some numerical comparisons may indeed represent true associations but not reach statistical significance. By the standards of scientific reporting, these associations would not qualify as study findings. However, understanding the limitations of inadequate statistical power and the importance of many different studies observing the same nonstatistically significant patterns, we choose to call attention to some of the observed data.

Of the eight rate ratios noted at the 40 percent increased or decreased risk thresholds, seven were elevated. If we eliminate the two “all participants” relative risks, considering them duplicative of the boarder and nonboarder data, we still have five elevations out of the six independent rate ratios considered. One might entertain the possibility that this is a nonrandom pattern.

We note with interest the thyroid cancer risk ratios. First, thyroid cancer is known to be radiogenic. Second, it is rarely fatal, so the incidence of thyroid cancers would not be reflected in the mortality data on which this study is based. Third, because there are only nine thyroid cancer deaths identified among CROSSROADS participants and controls, statistical comparisons do not have the power to pick up a statistically significant difference. Yet, the risk estimate for participants relative to controls is the highest found in this study. As discussed in the preceding paragraph, however, chance cannot be eliminated as an explanation.

Other Models and Parameters Considered During Analysis

As mentioned in the opening section of this chapter, we considered—using all-cause mortality—various interactions and combinations of variables in the building of the statistical models upon which we based this report. Here, we describe attempts at modeling and decisions made regarding paygrade, age, and Engineering & Hull status, and the interactions of participant status with each of them.

We use age as an independent variable to adjust the data for variations in age in the study cohorts. We considered a model in which both age-at-shot and age-at-shot-squared were variables. The estimated parameter coefficient for the age-at-shot squared variable was not statistically significant; we did not include the squared term in the final models.

We examined all-cause mortality, all-cancer mortality, and leukemia mortality in models testing a range of time-related variables. Neither time-since-shot nor age-at-shot interacted with exposure variables (participant status, boarder status, Engineering & Hull assignment) to produce statistically significant or otherwise observable relationships. Using the LIFETEST program in SAS to analyze survival times in participants and controls, we looked at data by age-at-shot strata, again finding nothing statistically significant and observing nothing that seemed to indicate time-dependent differences between the participants and the controls.

We checked whether the use of imputed dates of birth might have affected the results. Chapter 9 describes the procedure we had followed to impute missing dates of birth, using matched rank and paygrade. The all-cause mortality model run without these imputed dates, thereby excluding those 1,447 records (and 186 deaths) from the analysis, did not reveal different information. See Table 11-13.

TABLE 11-12. Nonsignificant Risk Estimates from Tables 11-4 and 11-5 that Indicate (boldface*) at Least a 40 percent Excess or Deficit in Mortality

		A: Basic	B: Boarder Gradient	
Case Definition	No. of Deaths	All Participants	Nonboarding Participants	Boarding Participants
Thyroid cancer	9	**3.479 (0.720–16.81)**	**3.248 (0.628–16.80)**	**4.235 (0.593–30.24)**
Hodgkin's Disease	45	0.748 (0.415–1.347)	**0.536 (0.264–1.090)**	**1.444 (0.673–3.097)**
Liver cancer	55	**1.492 (0.866–2.572)**	**1.533 (0.866–2.712)**	1.355 (0.576–3.188)
Lymphosarcoma and reticulosarcoma	71	0.998 (0.627–1.591)	0.767 (0.449–1.313)	**1.787 (0.973–3.283)**

*In this table (distinct from earlier tables) the **boldfaced** values mark rate ratios ≥1.4 or ≤0.6.

TABLE 11-13. All-Cause Mortality Rate Ratios, Including and Excluding Records with Imputed Dates of Birth

	Model A[a]	Model B[b]	
Imputed Dates of Birth	All Participants	Nonboarding Participants	Boarding Participants
Including imputed DOBs	**1.046 (1.020–1.074)**[c]	**1.043 (1.015–1.073)**	**1.057 (1.014–1.102)**
Excluding imputed DOBs	**1.051 (1.024–1.079)**	**1.052 (1.023–1.082)**	**1.049 (1.006–1.094)**

[a]Model A compares all participants to all nonparticipants, adjusting for paygrade and age at shot.
[b]Model B uses gradient of potential exposure and compares nonboarding participants and boarding participants to all nonparticipants (controls), adjusting for paygrade and age at shot.
[c]**Boldface** represents statistical significance at $p < 0.05$ level.

We looked at various ways of handling *occupation, paygrade,* and potential interactions of *paygrade and participant status and boarder status and Engineering & Hull.* These did not yield informative results; the earlier described models were not changed.

STANDARDIZED MORTALITY RATIOS

Analysis of the data using standardized mortality ratios (SMRs) yields results consonant with the findings we have discussed thus far in this section. Please refer to Chapter 8 and Appendix C for rationale and detailed results. In this study for the Navy, all-cause SMRs were 0.8715 for participants and 0.8322 for controls. For all malignancies and leukemias, they were, respectively, 0.8196 and 1.004 for participants and 0.8156 and 1.079 for controls.

DISCUSSION RELATING THESE FINDINGS TO THOSE OF SIMILAR STUDIES

The data and findings we present in this report of CROSSROADS mortality are consistent with findings of earlier studies of nuclear test participants.

Findings in Other Studies of Atomic Veterans

In 1988, Darby and colleagues reported on a study of 22,347 men involved in the British nuclear test program from 1952 to 1967. The participants for the study were identified from a multitude of records by the British Ministry of Defense (MOD) and are distributed among the services as follows: 29 percent Navy, 27 percent Army, 40 percent Air Force, and another 4 percent civilian. In determining the completeness of the participant list, the investigators identified 2,121 "independent respondents" who were found through solicitation of sources apart from MOD (e.g., veterans' groups) and were verified as participants. Of these, 1,707 were found to be on the main study list, suggesting a completeness of 83 percent. Using only the main study list (MOD-generated), Darby et al. reported mortality of participants relative to controls of 1.01 (90% confidence interval, 0.95–1.07). However, when adjusted for the independent respondents who were not included in the main study, all-cause mortality increased to 1.05 (90% confidence interval, 0.97–1.13).

The CROSSROADS study differs from the Darby et al. study in that it covers only one nuclear test series whose nuclear detonations were completed within one month, six years before the beginning of the British testing period. The CROSSROADS cohort on which we base our analysis and conclusions is entirely Navy, but is 73 percent larger than the all-service Darby study cohort.

We estimate (see Appendix E) that the CROSSROADS participant roster is 93–99 percent complete. The apparent difference to Darby's 83 percent completeness is attributable mostly to differing U.S. and U.K. policies in assembling the lists. The identification methodology used by Nuclear Test Personnel Review (NTPR) includes self-identified participants who subsequently were verified as test participants through official records. The Darby list, however, is purely a MOD records-based compilation; it does not include self-identified participants. Thus, it is likely that our study is more similar to the Darby analysis with adjustments for missing participants than to the main study. Given that, our findings of a 1.046 (95% confidence interval, 1.02–1.074) relative risk for all-cause mortality in the participants over the controls seems to be in consonance with the Darby results.

In 1993, Darby et al. completed a second analysis of British atomic veterans that added an additional seven years of follow-up. At that time the relative risk for all-cause mortality was still near unity—0.99 (90% confidence interval, 0.95–1.05). In this study, Darby et al. did not report all-cause mortality for the main study adjusting for men not included in the main study. They did, however, study the "independent respondent" group separately and determined that the self-identified participants who were not found in the main MOD study list did have elevated mortality for both all causes and all cancers. This they attributed to a self-selection effect.

Watanabe, Kang, and Dalager (1995) reported finding increased relative risk for all-cause mortality in a study of 8,554 U.S. Navy personnel who participated in the HARDTACK nuclear test in 1958. Their study used the same NTPR database as this one, but dates of birth were not available for controls and many participants and relative risks were adjusted only for rank. Their comparison group of similar Navy nonparticipants numbered 14,625. In participants with an assigned dose of less than 2.5 mSv (0.25 rem), they observed a relative risk for all causes of death of 1.09 (95% CI, 0.98–1.21, n = 3345); for 2.5–10.0 mSv (0.251–1.00 rem), 1.08 (95% CI, 0.98–1.19, n = 4115); and for greater than 10 mSv (1.00 rem), 1.23 (95% CI, 1.04–1.45, n = 1094). Overall, the crude rate ratio for all-cause mortality in the study was 1.10 (95% CI, 1.02–1.19). The all-cause relative risk of 1.047 that we have observed is in consonance with these findings.

Selection Bias as an Explanation for Increased Participant All-Cause Mortality

Is it possible that a selection effect of having "independent respondents" included in our study by virtue of the NTPR process is alone responsible for our finding of a 5 percent increase in mortality for the participants? It is possible, but unlikely based on the discussion that follows. We have no data with which to determine exactly what fraction of the NTPR data set is self-identified. However, we estimate that we are missing between 1 and 7 percent of the participants. That allows us to estimate the magnitude of the self-identification problem.

Let us assume that all of the deaths among the "missing participants" would have appeared in the NTPR data set as a result of self-reporting after the onset of disease or from reporting by a member of the family during a posthumous filing of a claim for compensation. In other words, we assume our present number of deaths includes those deaths that would otherwise have gone uncaptured in a completely unbiased participant data set. Thus, our count of deaths would accurately reflect *all* participant deaths, but our count of participants would be low by 1–7 percent (approximately 400–2,700 people). If all these assumptions are true, our risk estimate for participants has used a correct numerator with a too-small denominator and is therefore biased upward. Were we to correct for that—by adding 400–2,700 people to the participant denominator and leaving the numerator as it is—we would get a 1–7 percent lower risk estimate. This is again consistent with Darby's findings.

The number of CROSSROADS personnel missed by the NTPR is thus critical to establishing the magnitude of the self-selection bias. In Appendix E we reported several estimates for missing participants. The highest of these was based on the match of our participant list to the National Association of Atomic Veterans (NAAV) list of CROSSROADS participants. All inexact matches were declared as missing participants, leading to a missing rate of 7 percent. If we adjust the crude mortality rate based on our assumptions above (i.e., that the deaths for the 7 percent missing participants are actually in our mortality count), the crude mortality in the participants drops by 7 percent, effectively wiping out the increased rate we have reported in the participants. The data on missing participants from the write-in study (see Appendix E) suggested a much lower missing rate of 3.7 percent; which would also reduce the crude participant death rate by 3.7 percent. After completing more detailed research on each of the suspected missing participants, we determined that from the NAAV list we would estimate only 1.5 percent participants to be missing and 1.1 percent to be missing if we use the write-in data. Given those estimates, our crude rates would drop only 1–2 percent in the participants if the self-selected deaths, who would otherwise have been missing, were removed. The latter two estimates are probably more accurate than the former two and suggest that, at most, half of the excess relative risk found in the participants for all-cause mortality would be attributable to self-selection in the NTPR process.

Furthermore, one would expect at least as large a self-selection effect on cancer mortality as on all-cause mortality. After all, preparation of claims for cancers thought to be a consequence of test participation would be one of the primary reasons a veteran would have for contacting the NTPR and becoming a member of the atomic veteran cohort. In this study, the all-malignancy relative risk, 1.014 (95% CI 0.962–1.068), was not statistically different from the all-cause relative risk, 1.046 (95% CI 1.020–1.074), and indeed the point estimate was smaller. Thus, the cancer mortality data do support the argument that the all-cause relative risk was elevated in the participants largely due to self-selection bias.

In summary, selection bias may have contributed to some degree to our finding of increased relative risk for all-cause mortality among CROSSROADS participants. Given the completeness of the participant roster and the lack of a concomitant increase in all-malignancy risk, however, it is unlikely that this bias accounts for all of the increase observed.

AVENUES OF FURTHER EXPLORATION

Because the value of the work invested in this study of CROSSROADS may not be fully apparent, we close this report with our views of what has been accomplished and what can still be accomplished using this extraordinary database. We now have a dataset with the records of 80,000 individuals who served in the U.S. Navy in 1946. Most typographic and administrative recording errors have been corrected; missing data have been, when appropriate, estimated, with documentation to provide justification; the participant cohort is 93–99 percent complete; vital status follow-up across almost 50 years is around 90 percent—this is approaching, in fact, a total follow-up rather than a study sample.

Many conceptual and practical limitations recede with complete mortality ascertainment in a cohort. At some point, regrettably, all of the participants at CROSSROADS will have died. Even if that is another 50 years from now, we should maintain the data resource and update vital status follow-up. A study of the complete mortality experience of the CROSSROADS participant and comparison group cohorts would carry minimal marginal cost relative to what has been invested so far. We hope that resources could be provided to maintain, permanently document, and update this database.

Questions that might suitably be asked of these data—with supplemental information collected as necessary—are:

- What more can we learn about the associations military paygrade and rank have with mortality? Does short-term versus career military participation provide clues? To what extent might career-mortality associations be the result of selection decisions about military service, career success and promotion, or occupational exposures?
- What more can we learn about the mortality experience of the Army and Marine personnel who participated in Operation CROSSROADS? Using a larger sample, an IOM committee and staff are now building a comparison group to study the military participants in five other U.S. atmospheric test series.

It would be informative to consider test-specific duties as well as rank/occupation of Army and Marine personnel in building an appropriate comparison cohort, as the CROSSROADS study was able to do in significant numbers for Navy personnel.

- What can we learn by analyzing, in addition to the underlying causes used in this report, the associated causes of death listed on death certificates for the CROSSROADS participants and controls? Might there be clues to reporting bias? Might there be information that gives us a better understanding of the morbidity experience of these individuals? Finally, can the contribution of a self-selection bias in the participant cohort be quantified? And, how best can we control for it in ongoing and future studies of atomic veterans?

12

Conclusions

SUMMARY OF FINDINGS

Among Navy personnel, the primary analysis group for this study, we found that participants at the CROSSROADS nuclear test experienced higher mortality than a comparable group of nonparticipating military controls. The increase in all-cause mortality was 4.6 percent (relative risk [RR] = 1.046, 95% confidence interval, 1.020–1.074) and was statistically significant ($p < 0.001$).[27] For malignancies, the elevation of mortality was lower—RR = 1.014 (0.96–1.068)—and was not statistically significant ($p = 0.26$). Similarly, leukemia mortality RR was elevated to 1.020 (0.75–1.39), but not significantly ($p = 0.90$) and by less than all-cause mortality. The increase in all-cause mortality did not appear to concentrate in any of the disease groups we considered. Of the 44 other specific cancers and disease categories we examined, there were no statistically significant increases in mortality. The overall elevation of mortality rate ratios for malignancies and leukemias in the participants were not statistically significant and, in fact, were lower than for many other causes of death.

Navy mortality due to all malignancies and leukemia did not vary substantially among our exposure surrogate groups (i.e., those who boarded target ships after a detonation vs. those who did not, and those enlisted

[27] All statistical tests are two-sided.

Participants who boarded target ships were thought to be a more highly exposed than the rest of the participant group. Relative to the controls (nonparticipating comparison group), boarding participants experienced a 5.7 percent increase in all-cause mortality, RR equal to 1.057 (1.014–1.10), p = 0.0093, whereas the nonboarders (less exposed participant group) experienced a 4.3 percent increase (RR = 1.043 [1.015–1.073], p = 0.0028). Aside from all-cause mortality, risks for boarding participants did not significantly exceed those for controls for any of the disease categories, and risks relative to controls were similar for boarding and nonboarding participants. The increase in risk for all-malignancies among the participants was 2.6 percent (RR = 1.026 [0.94–1.12], p = 0.55) for boarders and 1 percent (RR = 1.010 [0.95–1.068], p = 0.73) for nonboarders. For leukemia, the increase in mortality risk for boarders was, 0.7 percent (RR = 1.007 [0.61–1.66], p = 0.98) and for nonboarders, 2.4 percent (RR = 1.024 [0.737–1.422], p = 0.89). In all cases the 95% confidence intervals overlap, suggesting the difference between boarders and nonboarders could well be due to chance.

Those Navy participants holding an Engineering & Hull (E&H) occupational specialty were thought to be more highly exposed to radiation than their non-E&H counterparts. However, the E&H participants had essentially the same risk of mortality from all causes as non-E&H participants (RR = 0.99 [0.95–1.038], p = .81). For all malignancies and leukemias, the rate ratios were somewhat higher, 1.051 [0.97–1.14] and 1.51 [0.94–2.44] respectively, but both could be attributed to chance (p = 0.25 and 0.088 respectively). Risk ratios for leukemia and malignancies among E&H controls showed a similar elevation relative to non-E&H controls, suggesting that a factor specifically associated with CROSSROADS was not likely to have been the cause.

These findings do not support a hypothesis that exposure to ionizing radiation was the cause of increased mortality among CROSSROADS participants. Had radiation been a significant contributor to increased risk of mortality, we should have seen significantly increased mortality due to malignancies, particularly leukemia, in participants thought to have received higher radiation doses relative to participants with lower doses and to unexposed controls. We did not observe any such effects. We note, however, that this study was neither intended not designed to be an investigation of low-level radiations effects, per se, and it should not be interpreted as such.

In comparing the findings and methods employed in this study with those of other investigations of atomic veteran mortality, we have identified a possible self-selection bias in the participant cohort: participants who died of a disease (particularly cancer) may have been more likely than healthy participants to have identified themselves to the NTPR, and hence become a part of this study. Such a bias would have resulted in an apparent increase in death rates among the participants. We do not have data with which to make a good quantitative estimate of this potential bias. However, the roster of participants is nearly complete, and mortality from all malignancies and leukemia was lower, not higher, than the increase in all-cause mortality. These factors suggest that a self-selection bias was not entirely responsible for the finding of increased all-cause mortality in study participants.

We believe that the elevated risk of all-cause mortality in CROSSROADS participants relative to a comparable military comparison group is probably the result of two factors. The first is an unidentified factor, other than radiation, associated with participation in, or presence at, the CROSSROADS test. The second is a self-selection bias within the participant roster. However, the relative contributions of these two explanations cannot be accurately determined within available resources for this project.

References

Beebe GW and Simon AH. Ascertainment of mortality in the U.S. veteran population. *American Journal of Epidemiology* 89:636–643, 1969.

Bradley D. *No Place to Hide 1946/1984.* Hanover, NH: University Press of New England, 1948, 1983.

Caldwell GG, Kelley DB, and Heath CW. Leukemia among participants in military maneuvers at a nuclear bomb test. A preliminary report. *Journal of the American Medical Association* 244:1575–1578, 1980.

Caldwell, GG, Kelley DB, and Zack M. Mortality and cancer frequency among military nuclear test (SMOKY) participants, 1957 through 1979. *Journal of the American Medical Association* 250:620–624, 1983.

Campbell R. NAAV's mortality study of civilian test site workers and Ohio uranium plant workers verifies previous findings of premature death rates of military personnel exposed to ionizing radiation. *Atomic Veteran's Newsletter* 16(1), Spring 1994.

Cox DR. Regression models and life-tables (with discussion). *Journal of the Royal Statistical Society* Series B 34:187–220, 1972.

Darby SC, Kendall GM, Fell TP, et al. A summary of mortality and incidence of cancer in men from the United Kingdom who participated in the United Kingdom's atmospheric nuclear weapon tests and experimental programmes. *British Medical Journal* 296:332, 1988.

Darby SC, Kendall GM, Fell TP, et al. *Mortality and Cancer Incidence 1952–1990 in UK Participants in the UK Atmospheric Nuclear Weapon Tests and Experimental Programmes.* Report No. NRPB-R266, National Radiological Protection Board, Oxon, United Kingdom, 1993.

Darby SC, Kendall GM, Fell TP, et al. Further follow up of mortality and incidence of cancer in men from the United Kingdom who participated in the United Kingdom's atmospheric nuclear weapon tests and experimental programmes. *British Medical Journal* 307:1530–1535, 1993.

DNA (Defense Nuclear Agency). *Operation CROSSROADS—1946.* Report No. DNA-6032F, Alexandria, VA: Defense Nuclear Agency, 1984.

DNA (Defense Nuclear Agency). Operation CROSSROADS. Fact Sheet, Public Affairs Office, Washington, DC: Defense Nuclear Agency, April 5, 1984.

Federal Register (6-1) Vol. 54 No 118, p. 26029, Wednesday June 21, 1989 Rules and regulations.

Gelband H. A discussion of questions about the 1985 NAS report *Mortality of Nuclear Weapons Test Participants.* Office of Technology Assessment, U.S. Congress, Washington DC, August 1992.

GAO (General Accounting Office). *Mortality Study of Atmospheric Nuclear Test Participants is Flawed.* Report to the Chairman, Committee on Veterans' Affairs, U.S. Senate, Report No. GAO/RCED-92-182. Washington DC: GAO, August 1992.

Gunderson EKE. Organizational and environmental influences on health and performance. Report 76-39, Naval Medical Research and Development Command, Department of the Navy, 1976.

Helmkamp JC and Bone CM. Hospitalizations for accidents and injuries in the U.S. Navy. I. Duty station assignment and duty status. Report No. 85-5, Naval Health Research Center, Naval medical Research and Development Command, Bethesda, MD, 1985a.

Helmkamp JC and Bone CM. Hospitalizations for accidents and injuries in the U.S. Navy. II. External cause of accident, duty station assignment, and level of seniority. Report No. 85-8, Naval Health Research Center, Naval Medical Research and Development Command, Bethesda, MD, 1985b.

Helmkamp JC and Colcord CL. Hospitalization rates among selected Navy enlisted occupations by age, education and paygrade. Report No. 84-34, Naval Health Research Center, Naval Medical Research and Development Command, Bethesda, MD, 1984.

Ingram DD and Makuc DM. Statistical issues in analyzing the NHANES. Epidemiologic Follow-up Study. (Vital and health statistics. Series 2. Data evaluation and methods research, No. 121.) Hyattsville, MD: DHHS publication No. (PHS) 94-1395, 1994.

IOM (Institute of Medicine). Review of the dosimetry data available in the Nuclear Test Personnel Review (NTPR) program. An interim letter report of the Committee to Study the Mortality of Military Personnel Present at Atmospheric Tests of Nuclear Weapons to the Defense Nuclear Agency. May 15, 1995a.

IOM (Institute of Medicine). *Adverse Reproductive Outcomes in Families of Atomic Veterans: The Feasibility of Epidemiologic Studies.* Washington, DC: National Academy Press, 1995b.

NCI (National Cancer Institute). Updated U.S. Mortality Rates (December 1993). In Information Management Services, Inc., Rockville, MD, letter dated February 1, 1995.

NCHS (National Center for Health Statistics). *Health, United States, 1991.* Hyattsville, MD: Public Health Service, 1992.

NRC (National Research Council). Committee on the Biological Effects of Ionizing Radiations). *Health Effects of Exposure to Low Levels of Ionizing Radiation* (BEIR V). Washington, DC: National Academy Press, 1990.

Naus JI. *Data Quality Control and Editing.* New York: Marcel Dekker, 1975.

NAVSPERS. Career pattern of the United States Navy. NAVPERS-NRB-52084-7 Feb 1949-50M (B91-0).

Page WF. VA mortality reporting for World War II Army veterans (letter). *American Journal of Public Health* 82(1):124–125, 1992.

Page WF, Braun MM, and Caporaso NE. Ascertainment of mortality in the U.S. veteran population: World War II twins. *Military Medicine* 160:351–355, 1995.

Pierce DA, Yukiko S, Preston KL, Vaeth M, and Mabuchi K. Studies of the Mortality of Atomic Bomb Survivors, Report 12, Part I. Cancer:1950–1990. *Radiation Research* 146:1-37, 1996

Preston DL, Lubin JH, Pierce DA, and McConney ME. *Epicure: User's Guide.* Seattle, WA: HiroSoft International Corporation, 1988–93.

Robinette CD, Jablon S, and Preston TL. *Studies of Participants in Nuclear Tests.* National Research Council. Washington, DC: National Academy Press, 1985.

Rockefeller JD IV. Opening statement, November 14, 1985 hearing before the Committee on Veterans' Affairs, United States Senate. *Oversight on Issues Pertaining to Veterans' Exposure to Ionizing Radiation.* S. Hrg. 99-542. Washington DC: U.S. Government Printing Office, 1986.

SAS Institute Inc. SAS Technical Report P-229, *SAS/STAT Software: Changes and Enhancements, Release 6.07.* Cary, ND: SAS Institute, Inc., 1992.

Shigematsu I, Ito C, Kamada N, et al. *Effects of A-Bomb Radiation on the Human Body.* Tokyo: Bunkodo, 1995.

Stender WW and Walker E. The National Personnel Records Center fire: a study in disaster. *The American Archivist* 57:521, 1974.

UNSCEAR. *Sources and Effects of Ionizing Radiation.* 1994 Report to the General Assembly with Scientific Annexes. New York: United Nations, 1994.

Upton AC. Radiation. In *Cancer Medicine* (second edition), JF Holland and E Frei III, editors. Philadelphia: Lea & Febiger, 1982.

VA (Department of Veterans Affairs). Letter from Mr. J. Gary Hickman, Director, Compensation and Pension Service to Mr. D. M. Schaeffer, NTPR program, Defense Nuclear Agency, 7 July 1993.

Watanabe KK, Kang HK, and Dalager NA. Cancer mortality risk among military participants of a 1958 atmospheric nuclear weapons test. *American Journal of Public Health*, 85:523, 1995.

World Health Organization. *International Classification of Diseases, 9th Revision, Clinical Modification (ICD-9-CM).* In *The Educational Annotation of ICD-9-CM* (4th edition), CD Puckett, editor. Reno, NV: Channel Publishing, 1995.

A

National Association of Atomic Veterans (NAAV) Medical Survey

"NAAV Data Center"
2310 Apollo Way, Mesquite, Texas 75150-5329
FAX: 214/216-1838

March 9, 1995

J.C. Johnson, Ph.D., CHP
National Academy of Sciences
Institute of Medicine, Medical Follow-Up Agency
2101 Constitution Avenue
Washington, D.C. 20418

Dear Dr. Johnson,

In reply to your letter of March 7, 1995, requesting registration criteria utilized to select Atomic Veterans to be placed on the NAAV Registry, the following is submitted for your information.

Since the formation of NAAV in 1978, various personnel have attempted to compile data an the medical problems faced by veterans who participated during the period of "Atmosphere Testing". Additionally, those veterans who were POW's and those veterans who were occupation troops near Hiroshima and Nagasaki have been included with the test personnel. Together these veterans have come to be known as "Atomic Veterans".

During my tenure as the National Commander and NAAV Board Chairman from 1986 through 1989, I discovered records and files of various Medical Surveys which had been conducted by NAAV. In 1992, we started collecting these survey forms in one file location, cataloging them by Test Series, and entering the data from these survey forms into a computer data base (FileMaker II and then FileMaker Pro) where the various categories of information are sortable into desired and usable data. Our present Medical Survey Questionnaire was developed at that time. Each new member since mid 1992 has been requested to complete a survey form for our records. Presently, I receive an average about 10 of these survey forms each week.

The following sources of information are utilized to compile information on each veteran listed in the NAAV Medical Survey Data Registry:

a. A NAAV Medical Survey Questionnaire completed by the veteran or his widow. Specifically the years 1980, 1983, 1985-1986, 1992-1995. Many questionnaires are accompanied by copies of orders, DD-214 forms, discharge papers, doctors and hospital reports, VA documents, and DNA correspondence and/or registry forms.

b. Correspondence files containing letters of inquires from veterans, their widows or children along with discharge documents, copies of orders, media articles, Guinea Pig Certificates, Letters of Commendation, VA documents and claim forms, etc.

c. Information furnished by widows, ie, Death Certificates, DD-214 Forms, discharge papers, newspaper articles, VA documents and claim forms, etc.

All of this information is being sorted, cataloged, and entered into the NAAV computer data base to provide NAAV management with facts and figures usable in our efforts to "Obtain Simple Justice".

In addition to Test Personnel, we are collecting Medical Survey information on other classes of exposed veterans. What could be termed the second generation Atomic Veteran. Personnel involved in Broken Arrow incidents, nuclear submarine crewmen, nuclear weapons handlers and custodians, etc. I have about 150 of this category so far.

We don't usually hear from a veteran until he connects in his mind that his health problems might be related to his exposure. Also widows discover who we are and contact us concerning their husbands involvement in nuclear testing. Since we operate on members dues and member donations only, we have little money to advertise the plight of atomic veterans and their families and even less to utilize on a project such as this registry. This registry is my labor of love for the last three years with a little help from my friends. If any of you fat cats have any grant money laying around, I could put it to good use for stationary supplies, postage, data entry, and phone bills.

The data furnished you recently is but a snap shot of our registry. By the end of this year we hope to have available on the NAAV Registry most of the health survey information collected by NAAV on Atomic Veterans over the past 18 years. At that point we will add Correspondence file and data received from Widows to the registry.

Unfortunately, much information has been lost because of veteran deaths and by a government who covered up individual's stupidity because they put security before compassion, fear of lawsuits above individual suffering, and official's pride and ego over truth.

I am personally very pleased that the data transfer was successful. I regret that not all of the information on Crossroad veterans is completed as I still have to enter information on personnel from the Radiological Safety Section and the Ammunition Disposal Teams during Operation Crossroads. Perhaps you will accept and update sometime in the future.

I hope that some time in the future I might be able to study your report and conclusions. Please feel free to call on me for any assistance I might be able to furnish the Crossroads study or the Five Tests study.

I remain,

Sincerely,

Boley H. Caldwell III
LTC(Ret) U.S. Army

NATIONAL ASSOCIATION
OF
ATOMIC VETERANS

Medical History & Data Questionnaire

When Completed, Please Return to
NAAV, P.O. BOX 4424
SALEM, MA 01970

From time to time it is necessary for NAAV to provide statistical medical information on Atomic Veterans to our members, the news media, to Congress in support of legislation, the Department of Veterans' Affairs, the Department of Justice, and other government agencies. Without having a readily available medical data base on you, your children and grandchildren, we can not properly represent you.The last up date of our data files was in 1986, therefore we are requesting Atomic Veterans to complete this questionnaire and return it to NAAV as soon as possible.

If the individual veteran is deceased, it is particularly important that this questionnaire be completed as accurately as possible by a relative or friend. If possible, please enclose a copy of the Death Certificate with this completed questionnaire.

No information released will be in violation of the "Privacy Act". For the most part the information released is in the form of statistics. Most questions are straight forward but if you have a question please do not hesitate to contact us.

IMPORTANT: Please read the following statement, sign and date on the lines provided. Your signature is required. Thank you.

I understand that this information is needed so that NAAV can help with problems that I may have and so that certain medical research authorities, with NAAV's approval, may pursue medical problems of importance to all Atomic Veterans. The information I provide may be used by NAAV to advance the cause of the Atomic Veterans.

____
(Signature)

____
(Date)

PART I: Personal Information

1. Your Name - as spelled while in the military (or as a civilian employee).
First:__________ Middle: __________ Last: __________
2. Your address where you can be contacted
Address: ____________________
City: __________ State: ________ ZIP Code: ________
3. Telephone Number: (Include Area Code) (____) ____ - ______
4. Birth Date: Month ____ Day ____ Year ____
5. Sex: Male _ Female _ Race: ______ 6. SSN: ___-__-_____
7. Branch of Service: _______ 8. Military Service No: _________
9. Dates of Military Service: From __________ to __________
10. Rank at time of test __________
11. Rank at time of discharge __________
12. D.V.A. Claim No: _________ 11. Claim Results: _________
13. Name of friend or relative who would know your address, should you move.
Name: ______________ Telephone No: (___) ____ - _____
Address: ____________________
City: __________ State: ________ ZIP Code: ________

PART II: Atomic/Nuclear Test Participation

14. Which of the following series of tests did you participate in?

_ 1945 Alamogordo	_ 1945 Hiroshima	_ 1945 Nagasaki
_ 1946 Crossroads	_ 1948 Sandstone	_ 1951 Ranger
_ 1951 Greenhouse	_ 1951 Buster/Jangle	_ 1952 Tumbler/Snapper
_ 1952 Ivy	_ 1953 Upshot/Knothole	_ 1954 Castle
_ 1955 Teapot	_ 1955 Wigwam	_ 1956 Redwing
_ 1957 Plumbbob	_ 1958 Plumbbob	_ 1958 Hardtack I, II
_ 1958 Argus I, II, III	_ 1961 Nougat	_ 1962 Dominic I, II
_ 1979 Enewitok Cleanup		

_ Other Tests: Dates__________ Name______________
Description____________________
15. Ship/Unit/Duties during tests.____________________

Please use additional sheets of paper to give full details for each shot and exposure to ionizing radiation in activities other than testing.
16. Dates in the test area(s). (M/D/Y) From: ________ to ________
17. Were you issued: Film Badge Yes _ No _ ; Dosimeter Yes _ No _
Protective Clothing Yes ___ No ___; Radiac Meter Yes ___ No ___.
18. Approximate total time of your exposure to radiation _____(days)

Part III: Health/ Medical Information.

19. During the first six weeks after exposure, did you suffer any of the following medical problems? Please check as many as apply. Check twice if you received medical treatment for any of the conditions listed:

__ Rashes __ Nausea __ Vomiting __ Redness of Skin
__ Loss of Hair __ Diarrhea __ Nerves __ Fatigue/Apathy
__ Bleeding gums __ Other ____________

20. If you were treated for any medical problems during the first few weeks after the test detonation(s), If you can, please name the Location/Unit/Doctor/Medical Problem, etc. Please give all the particulars you can remember: ____________

21. Do you currently have, or have you had in the past, any of the following medical problems:

__ Cataracts __ Loss of Teeth __ Lymphoma __ Diabetes __ Sterility
__ Polycythemia Vera __ Multiple Myeloma __ Cancer of Bile Ducts
__ Heart Attacks(s) (No. __) __ Cancer of Thyroid __ Breast Cancer
__ Leukemia __ Cancer of Pharynx __ Cancer of Small Intestine
__ Heart Surgery __ Cancer of Esophagus __ Cancer of Pancreas
__ Cancer of Stomach __ Cancer of Gall Bladder __ Bone Cancer
__ Primary Liver Cancer __ Chromosomal Damage __ Cancer of Testes

22. Have you had a physical examination at a D.V.A. medical facility in accordance with Public Law 97-72 ? Yes __ No __

23. Do you receive benefits under:
Public Law 100-321 ? Yes __ No __ or (From D.V.A.)
Public Law 98-542 ? Yes __ No __ or (From D.V.A.)
Public Law 101-426? Yes __ No __ (From Dept of Justice)

24. D.V.A. hospital you presently are being treated / plan to be treated:

Name ____________
Address ____________
City ____________ State ________ ZIP Code ________

PART IV: Family Information

25. __ Married __ Widowed __ Divorced __ Single
26. Wife's name: ____________
27. Number of children _____ Number of Grandchildren _____
28. Please furnish information on any child or grandchild who has health problems which may relate to your exposure to ionizing radiation. (Continusd on page 4.)

PART V: Health Problems of Children and Grandchildren that may be due to veteran's exposure to ionizing radiation. Encircle S(Son), D(Daughter), GS (Grandson), GD (Granddaughter). Check illnesses.

A. Syndromes S D GS GD ____ Down's S D GS GD ____ Turner's ____ Others S D GS GD

B. Diseases that may be due to damage to Veteran's Reproductive System
S D GS GD ___ Multiple Sclerosis S D GS GD ____ Cystic Fibrosis Others S D GS GD

C. Birth Defects(Congenital Deformations).
Abnormal Growths. Describe S D GS GD

Others: S D GS GD
D. Learning Disabilities S D GS GD ____ Mental Retardation
S D GS GD ___ Slow Learner S D GS GD ____ Low IQ Others S D GS GD

E. Health Problems Same As Fathers or Grandfathers. Refer to p. 3.
__ Cataracts __ Loss of Teeth __ Lymphoma __ Diabetes __ Sterility
__ Polycythemia Vera __ Multiple Myeloma __ Cancer of Bile Ducts
__ Heart Attacks(s) (No. __) __ Cancer of Thyroid __ Breast Cancer
__ Leukemia __ Cancer of Pharynx __ Cancer of Small Intestine
__ Heart Surgery __ Cancer of Esophagus __ Cancer of Pancreas
__ Cancer of Stomach __ Cancer of Gall Bladder __ Bone Cancer
__ Primary Liver Cancer __ Chromosomal Damage __ Cancer of Testes
__ Others ____________

PART VI: Additional Information and Comments.

B

Participant Description
(DNA Memorandum dated July 11, 1994)

EXPLANATORY MEMORANDUM

BACKGROUND

CROSSROADS was a two-shot atmospheric nuclear test series conducted at Bikini Atoll during July and August 1946. The first test (Shot ABLE) was a device dropped on 1 July 1946 from an aircraft and exploded at an altitude of 520 feet over an array of target ships. The second test (Shot BAKER) was detonated on 25 July 1946, 90 feet below the water's surface amongst an array of target ships.

Two hundred forty-two ships participated in Operation CROSSROADS. Over 39,300 U.S. Navy personnel have been identified as having participated in the operation. The ships that participated can be divided into three categories: support ships, remanned target ships and unremanned target ships. Support ships were present at the test site at some time during the operational period, but were not in the target area at the time of the shots. Remanned target ships were ships that were present in the target area at the time of the shots. The crews for these ships were evacuated to support ships at the time of the detonations. The damage and contamination of these ships was such that it was determined they could be remanned by their crews after the detonations. The third category of ships, unremanned target ships, were also present in the target area at the time of the detonations. However, their crews, which had been evacuated to support ships, could not permanently return to their home ships because the ships had either sunk or were too severely damaged or contaminated to be remanned. Most of the crews of the unremanned target ships were shipped as passengers back to Kwajalein, Pearl Harbor and California west coast ports. About 10% of the crews for the unremanned target ships were assigned as replacement crewmembers of support ships. The three categories of ships included many types such as battleships, cruisers, destroyers, oilers, troop transports, aircraft carriers, submarines, patrol, supply, salvage, yard and utility ships.

OPERATIONAL PERIOD AND OPERATIONAL AREA

The Operational Area for this data collection effort is defined as Bikini Atoll. The Operational Period is defined as 1 July 1946 through 31 August 1946. All service members who were present in the Operational Area for any time during the Operational Period qualify for participation. Some personnel at Kwajalein and Enewetak also qualify as participants because they were at those locations to support the operation. The Post Operational Period for CROSSROADS extends from 1 September 1946 through 28 February 1947.

The activities of operational participants are documented throughout the Post Operational period to the extent possible.

SOURCES OF PARTICIPANT INFORMATION

The participants were identified from multiple sources such as service personnel records, unit diaries, ship deck logs, ship/unit muster rolls, ship/unit officer lists, unit histories, morning reports and operation participant listings. Great effort was expended to recover all relevant participation records. The quality, content and completeness of these records varies. The Army records are almost wholly insufficient to completely track participants. Most Army personnel arrived and departed by aircraft and there are no aviation records available to document arrival and departure dates. Army personnel also performed duties ashore at Bikini; however, available records do not document the specific activities of individuals ashore so these periods cannot be accounted for. Small segments of records have never been recovered and some units were so small that they never maintained individual records, e.g., small Navy vessels, such as "yard" craft with small crews, never maintained deck logs or crew lists.

Despite the great effort made to identify all CROSSROADS participants it is clear from the absence of complete records that not all participants have been found. "Staff Afloat" personnel aboard Navy ships were commonly not named and therefore not identifiable. This database is comprehensive in that every major participation element has been included but it has not been possible to identify all individual participants because of the inadequacies of the records.

TRACKING OF PARTICIPANTS

Units that entered the operational area prior to the first shot day generally have a participation start date of 1 July 1946. Units that entered the operational area after the first shot and during the operational period have a participation start date that corresponds to their actual date of arrival. During the operational period large-scale permanent and temporary transfers of personnel (mostly sailors) among the participating ships often occurred. The ships involved had differing levels of contamination which required that the sailors' service be tracked through all transfers among multiple ships. The periods of time spent aboard various ships are listed sequentially in the database. Where gaps in dates appear, they generally indicate a period of unknown location, either ashore or aboard an unidentified ship. Where possible, all sailors were tracked throughout their participation in the operational area at least to the point where they departed the ship that transported them from the operational area. Sailors who are not shown on available records to have departed their ship before its radiological clearance are assumed to have remained aboard to that date (generally late fall or early 1947) at which time their participation terminated as well as their dose accrual.

REFINEMENT OF THE INITIAL DATA BASE

In the initial data collection effort for this project over 2,500 sailors had incomplete names and were missing other essential data such as service numbers and rate/ratings. Through an extensive effort which involved ordering over 600 personnel records from the National Personnel Records Center in St. Louis, MO and multiple trips to the National Archives this number has been reduced to the absolute minimum.

Pseudo service numbers generated by a computer program have been assigned to participants for whom no service number could be found. These numbers can be identified by the prefix "DE" and/or the source code "23" The rate/rating is left blank for those participants for whom this information could not be found.

PARTICIPATION DATES AND DOSE RECONSTRUCTING

The start and stop participation dates and start and stop dose reconstruction dates will match for personnel who have been completely tracked. Some personnel have had "special" reconstructions computed as a result of VA claims or personal inquiries. These can generally be identified by the fact that they have reconstruction identification numbers in the database. Generic doses have been assigned to personnel of units that had special participation scenarios which made it impossible to document the activities of individual members of the unit. The participation and dose dates for personnel with generic doses commonly do not match. Personnel of the following units were assigned generic doses:

UNIT	MEAN DOSE
Det 1156 53rd Naval Const BN	1,140 mrem
Underwater Demolition Team 3	650 mrem
COMLCTGRU 21	1,350 mrem
COMLCTGRU 15	1,350 mrem

Doses were not computed for personnel whose participation status and activities could not be tracked/documented. These individuals often lack complete participation dates. The database may contain doses for these personnel but their source and accuracy have not been verified.

DOSE RECONSTRUCTION

The doses were reconstructed based on the participation dates and ships to which the sailors were assigned and the sailor's rate/rating. In about 80% of the cases the participants have been assigned High, Mean, and Low doses. The remaining 20% only have a Mean dose assigned. Generic doses have been assigned to certain groups of individuals who had common participation scenarios but whose individual activities could not be specifically evaluated. In cases where individuals were assigned film badges their recorded doses are shown in addition to their reconstructed ones.

ENGINEER RATINGS

Sailors who served below decks in engineering ratings (specialties) in close proximity to a ship's piping and evaporators had higher potential levels of radiation exposure, and thus received higher reconstructed doses than their non-engineering rated shipmates. Engineer rating are defined as: Carpenter Mates—CM, CM3, CM2, CM1, and CMC; Shipfitters—SF, SF3, SF2, SF1, and SFC; Water Tenders—WT, WT3, WT2, WT1, and WTC; Boilermakers—BT, BT3, BT2, BT1, and BTC; Fireman—F, FA, FN; and Machinist Mates—MM, MM3, MM2, MM1, and MMC. When engineers were in non-duty status i.e., sick, evacuation, transportation etc., their doses were computed at the non-engineering rate. The special provisions for engineers do not apply to submariners, seabees, and individuals with generic doses. The few sailors who started their participation as non-engineers and who were later promoted to an engineering rating during the participation period had their doses computed as non-engineers throughout their participation period.

SOURCE CODES

Data elements within the database are linked to source codes to identify the source of the data. For example: if a piece of data was obtained from a deck log, the deck log source code (29) is linked to that data element. Attached is a list of source codes authorized for use in the NTPR database.

PARTICIPATING UNIT/PERMANENT UNIT DATA

The database contains Participating and Permanent Unit fields for each participant. The Participating Unit data reflects where the individual was during the relevant period. Doses were computed on the basis of the Participating Unit data. The Permanent Unit data is irrelevant to a participant's dose.

COMMANDER JOINT TASK FORCE (CJTF-1) MEDICAL RESEARCH PERSONNEL, BOARDING TEAM AND RADSAFE TEAMS

Operation CROSSROADS was conducted under the command and control of CJTF-1. Approximately 1,100 personnel were assigned to CJTF-1. These personnel were assigned to conduct specialized functions such as instrumentation, oceanography, ordnance and electronic research. The nature of their duties required them to board target ships but dates and the ships boarded are not usually a matter of record. They have been tracked aboard their "home" and support ships and their doses have been computed on that basis. They can be identified in the database by the unit "CJTF 1" in the participating unit and/or permanent unit history data fields.

CJTF-1 personnel were also assigned as Boarding Teams and RADSAFE Team members. Their duties, to a far greater extent than other CJTF-1 personnel, required repeated and prolonged boarding of target ships. The doses for these individuals cannot be reliably reconstructed because of the absence of records documenting their presence aboard target ships. These individuals are identified as "Boarding Team" and "RADSAFE" in the participating unit field.

The duties of Medical Research personnel would have also required the boarding of target ships. However, their presence aboard the target ships is also not a matter of record. Their home ship was the USS BURLESON (APA 67). The reconstructed doses for these personnel are based on their time aboard BURLESON. These personnel are identified as "Medical Research" in the participating unit field.

C

Standardized Mortality Ratios

The commonly used standardized mortality ratio (SMR) succinctly compares the rates of death (or other endpoint of interest) of a cohort of interest with a (usually larger) stable, known population. The larger population rates help to stabilize estimates of rare disease or within sparse subject strata. SMRs also help put the relative rates in a perspective somewhat familiar to the reader. They allow comparisons, although informal, with other studies. For example, if group A risk is high relative to group B, SMRs using a population such as the U.S. males in 1950–1985 can shed light on whether that is because group A's rates are high or group B's are low.

We use the Epicure model AMFIT (Preston et al. 1988) and present the data in the same strata and outcome models that we use for the proportional hazard models, also using 95 percent confidence intervals. SMR analyses are multivariate in that they adjust for age and time period, using a weighted average of category-specific effects. A limitation to their use is that other variables are not included. Results are presented as a ratio of observed to expected, with 1 (or 100 if so standardized) representing equal rates, less than 1 if the observed rate is less than the expected rate, and greater than 1 if the expected exceeds the observed.

An oft-raised and truly considerable drawback to SMR use in studies of occupational-type exposures is the healthy worker—or soldier (sailor)—effect described in Chapter 3. In fact, an earlier mortality study of atmospheric nuclear tests and mortality (Robinette 1985) was criticized for using SMRs as its sole risk comparison. The study we report here was designed to include a military reference cohort to provide a finer comparison. The SMR comparison to the U.S. male population of the period under study adds, as mentioned above, a perspective that is useful as long as one keeps its limitations in mind.

The results of our SMR analysis are presented in the following pages by service and disease category. In the case of the Navy for all-cause and all-malignancy mortality (Tables C-1 to C-2), the cohort is subdivided into the seven analysis levels as described in Chapter 10. For Navy leukemias, there were insufficient numbers of cases to use the seven-level analysis. For leukemias (Table C-3), the SMR data are collapsed over ranks and presented by participant status, boarder status, and Engineering & Hull status. For the Army (Table C-4, including the Air Corps) and the Marines (Table C-5), no occupational information is available; therefore, SMRs are calculated for the service as a whole. The disease categories include:

- all-cause mortality,
- all-malignancy mortality, and
- all leukemia mortality.

The tabulations of mortality rates (U.S. white male) we used as a comparison standard in this SMR analysis included chronic lymphocytic leukemia (CLL), which is not thought to be radiogenic. Of these there were approximately equal numbers in the controls and participants (10 and 11 respectively). Because of its nonradiogenic nature, CLL was excluded in the primary analysis using the proportional hazards model (see Chapters 10 and 11).

TABLE C-1. Standardized Mortality Ratios for All Causes of Death in Navy Participants and Controls

		Observed	SMR	95% Conf. Intervals Lower	Upper
ENGINEERING AND HULL ENLISTED					
Junior	Boarder Participant	341	0.9089	0.8124	1.0050
	Control	973	0.8342	0.7818	0.8866
	Non-Boarding Participant	670	0.9099	0.8410	0.9788
Midlevel	Boarder Participant	247	0.8635	0.7558	0.9711
	Control	802	0.8739	0.8134	0.9344
	Non-Boarding Participant	650	1.0210	0.9423	1.0990
Senior	Boarder Participant	351	0.9747	0.8727	1.0770
	Control	1047	0.9231	0.8672	0.9791
	Non-Boarding Participant	771	0.8948	0.8317	0.9580
OFFICERS					
	Boarder Participant	255	0.5419	0.4754	0.6084
	Control	1213	0.5589	0.5274	0.5903
	Non-Boarding Participant	1008	0.5427	0.5092	0.5762
OTHER ENLISTED					
Junior	Boarder Participant	850	0.9866	0.9203	1.0530
	Control	3292	0.9062	0.8752	0.9371
	Non-Boarding Participant	2775	0.9708	0.9347	1.0070
Midlevel	Boarder Participant	405	1.0020	0.9041	1.0990
	Control	1890	0.8458	0.8077	0.8840
	Non-Boarding Participant	1899	0.9174	0.8761	0.9587
Senior	Boarder Participant	362	0.8899	0.7982	0.9816
	Control	1574	0.9198	0.8744	0.9652
	Non-Boarding Participant	1504	0.8921	0.847	0.9372
All Participants		12088	0.8715	0.8559	0.8870
All Controls		10791	0.8322	0.8165	0.8479

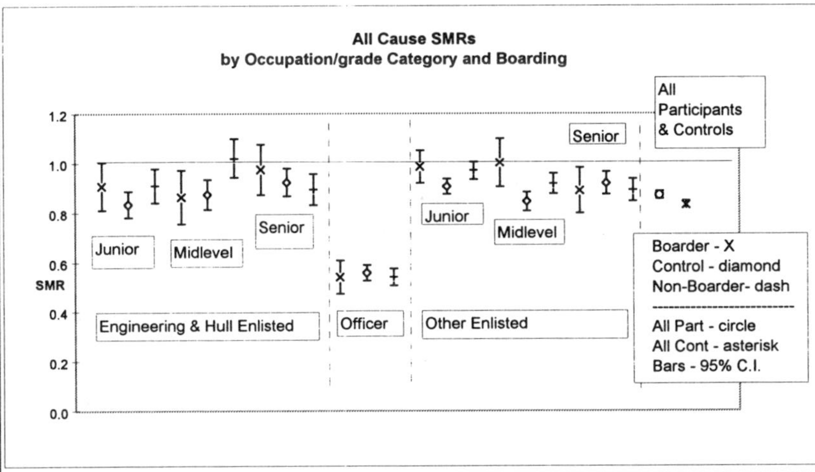

TABLE C-2. Standardized Mortality Ratios for All-Malignancy Deaths in Navy Participants and Controls

		Observed	SMR	95% Conf. Intervals Lower	Upper
ENGINEERING AND HULL ENLISTED					
Junior	Boarder Participant	81	0.8487	0.6639	1.0340
	Control	224	0.7505	0.6522	0.8488
	Non-Boarding Participant	169	0.9057	0.7692	1.0420
Midlevel	Boarder Participant	56	0.7576	0.5592	0.9561
	Control	217	0.9165	0.7945	1.0380
	Non-Boarding Participant	166	1.0130	0.8592	1.1680
Senior	Boarder Participant	82	0.9199	0.7208	1.119
	Control	288	1.0250	0.9068	1.1440
	Non-Boarding Participant	190	0.8875	0.7613	1.0140
OFFICERS					
	Boarder Participant	66	0.6072	0.4607	0.7537
	Control	301	0.5836	0.5177	0.6495
	Non-Boarding Participant	248	0.5755	0.5039	0.6471
OTHER ENLISTED					
Junior	Boarder Participant	182	0.8321	0.7112	0.9530
	Control	787	0.8477	0.7884	0.9069
	Non-Boarding Participant	627	0.8633	0.7957	0.9308
Midlevel	Boarder Participant	100	0.9660	0.7767	1.1550
	Control	464	0.8040	0.7308	0.8771
	Non-Boarding Participant	400	0.7505	0.6769	0.8240
Senior	Boarder Participant	100	0.9733	0.7825	1.1640
	Control	383	0.8929	0.8035	0.9823
	Non-Boarding Participant	375	0.8913	0.8011	0.9815
All Participants		2842	0.8196	0.7895	0.8497
All Controls		2664	0.8156	0.7846	0.8465

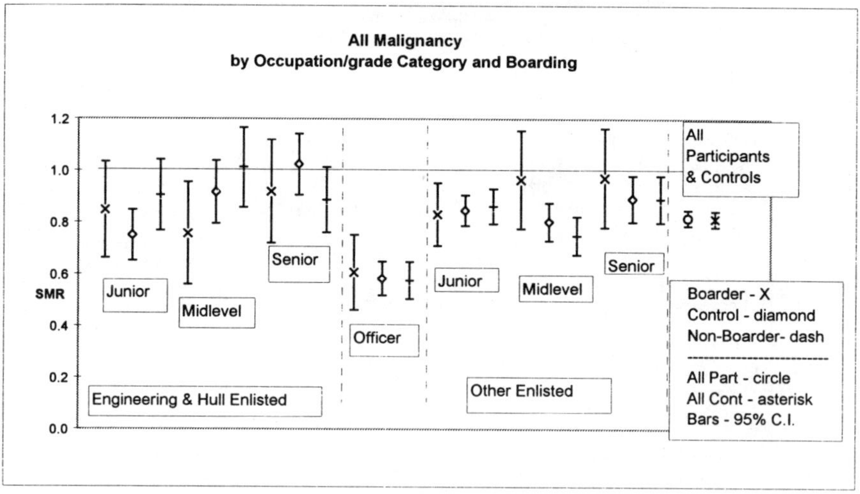

TABLE C-3. Standardized Mortality Ratios (SMR) for Leukemia (including CLL) for Navy Enlisted Personnel (n = 66,831)

	Engineering & Hull Status (E&H)	Boarding Status Nonboarders	Boarders
Control	Other enlisted	1.021 (0.7408–1.301) [51]	—
	E&H enlisted	1.403 (0.8922–1.913) [29] *	—
Participant	Other enlisted	0.8208 (0.5527–1.089) [36]	1.075 (0.4668–1.683) [12]
	E&H enlisted	1.654 (0.9924–2.316) [24]	0.9001 (0.1799–1.620) [6]

* Numbers of cases are shown in square brackets.

TABLE C-4. Standardized Mortality Ratios (SMR) for Army (including Army Air Corps, n = 6,482)

Case Definition	All Participants Deaths	SMR	All Controls Deaths	SMR
All Causes	1,192	0.6587 (0.6213–0.6961)	1,250	0.8662(0.8182–0.9142)
All Malignancies	261	0.6074 (0.5337–0.6811)	273	0.7789(0.6865–0.8713)
Leukemias	12	1.114 (0.4838–1.745)	8	0.9055(0.2780–1.533)

TABLE C-5. Standardized Mortality Ratios (SMR) for Marines (n = 1,137)

Case Definition	All Participants Deaths		All Controls Deaths	SMR
All Causes	173	0.8741 (0.7438–1.004)	174	0.8280 (0.7049–0.9510)
All Malignancies	47	0.9524 (0.6801–1.225)	31	0.5858 (0.3796–0.7921)
Leukemias	1	1.2781 (0*–2.316)	3	1.3599 (0*–4.703)

*Model yielded lower confidence limits of –0.7510 and –0.2903 respectively.

D

Radiation Doses for CROSSROADS Participants and Exposure Surrogate Groups

Although a recent Institute of Medicine (IOM 1995a) study found that Defense Nuclear Agency (DNA) dose data are unsuitable for dose-response analysis (see Chapter 8), a subsequent report (IOM 1995b) noted that these data may provide a rough estimate of the magnitude of doses received by the Atomic Veterans:

> Of 210,000 participating veterans, about 1,200 received doses that were estimated to exceed 50 mSv (5 rem), which is the present annual exposure limit set by the U.S. Nuclear Regulatory Commission for workers occupationally exposed to radiation. About 20,000 participants were assigned doses that exceed the more conservative annual occupational limit, 20 mSv (2 rem), proposed by the International Commission on Radiological Protection. A total of 0.07 percent of the doses exceeded 100 mSv (10 rem), while the average dose for the Atomic Veterans was 6 mSv (0.6 rem). Although the dose assigned to a given veteran might change with further study, the distribution of doses across the cohort is unlikely to change significantly. (p. 70)

According to DNA figures, the CROSSROADS participants received doses that were, on the whole, smaller than those of other nuclear test participants.

The IOM (1995a, p. 13) study also noted that, "Although there is anecdotal evidence that individual doses may have been greatly underestimated in individual cases, the overall tendency may have been to overestimate both external and internal doses." Even so, the doses of record for the CROSSROADS participants are comparable in magnitude and variability to the additional doses received in one decade by residents of the Rocky Mountain region as compared with those received by residents of the rest of the United States. The lifetime doses received by CROSSROADS participants are well within the range of lifetime doses to the U.S. population resulting from naturally occurring radiation sources.

It is conceivable that a subset of the CROSSROADS participants, because of their specialized training, may have pursued careers in radiation sciences either within the services or as civilians (e.g., as health physicists, nuclear reactor operators, or nuclear engineers). It is probable that this group accrued substantially higher radiation doses after CROSSROADS than during the test itself. We have no means of controlling for this possibility.

Although the radiation doses to the CROSSROADS cohort appear low, veterans have been vocal in their assertions that they are significantly below what they should be, based upon their firsthand observations of conditions at the test site. That makes it all the more desirable that this study base its analyses on exposure factors other than these dose estimates.

A summary of the DNA-assigned doses for the boarding and occupational specialty categories are shown in Figure D-1 and Table D-1. Again, note that these categories were derived independent of any dose information.

Figure D-1. Mean Doses (taken from DNA estimates) for Occupational Groups by their Status as Boarders or Nonboarders. See Chapter 8 for a description of the occupational categories.

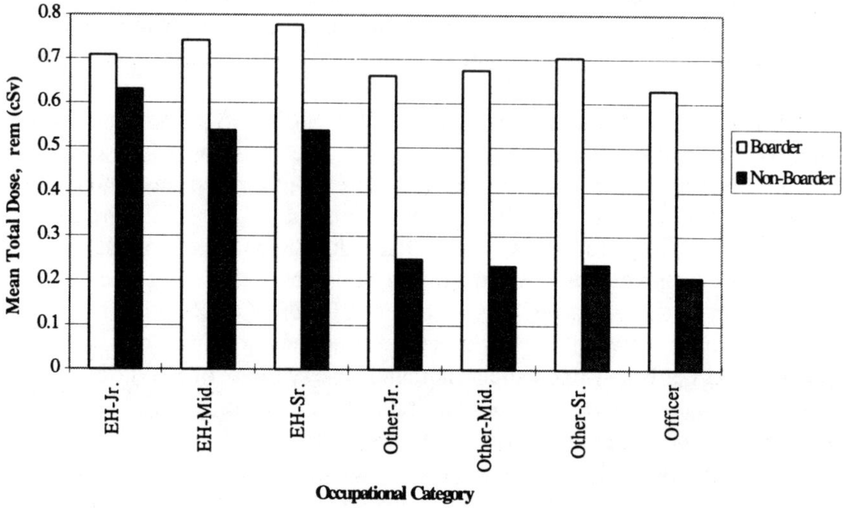

TABLE D-1. Tabulation of DNA Assigned Total Doses (rem (cSv)) by Study Grouping and Status as a Boarder or Nonboarder

	Mean		25%ile		50%ile		75%ile		Max.	
	Boarder	Non-boarder	Boarder	Non-boarder	Boarder	Non-boarder	Boarder	Non-boarder	Boarder	Non-boarder
EH-Jr.	0.709	0.631	0.362	0.418	0.706	0.689	1.001	0.783	2.356	2.548
EH-Mid	0.742	0.538	0.303	0.143	0.660	0.575	1.100	0.761	3.370	2.548
EH-Sr.	0.778	0.538	0.337	0.117	0.703	0.592	1.118	0.752	2.806	2.561
Other-Jr.	0.662	0.248	0.265	0.009	0.564	0.227	1.011	0.291	2.650	1.812
Other-Mid	0.674	0.234	0.259	0.001	0.586	0.213	1.001	0.277	3.130	2.609
Other-Sr.	0.704	0.236	0.262	0.001	0.586	0.212	1.013	0.277	3.245	2.251
Officer	0.629	0.208	0.233	0.002	0.477	0.199	1.001	0.272	2.920	3.732

E

Verification of Completeness and Accuracy of the Participant Roster

INTRODUCTION

Verification of the completeness and accuracy of the CROSSROADS participant file is particularly important to this study. In 1989, the Medical Follow-up Agency (MFUA) learned from the Nuclear Test Personnel Review (NTPR) that the participant roster provided for its 1985 "Five-Series" study of atomic veterans (NRC 1985) contained classification errors: approximately 15,000 nonparticipants were included as participants, while 28,000 actual participants were not included in the roster. These classification errors were discovered by NTPR in the process of updating its participant database after consolidating the individual service database into a single database in 1987. Subsequently, the General Accounting Office and the Office of the Technology Assessment (OTA) reported the origin and extent of the classification errors (GAO 1992; OTA 1992). The OTA report indicated that the number of misclassified individuals was smaller than originally indicated, but still significant, and recommended redoing that study.

NTPR delivered the first participant roster for CROSSROADS in 1986, well after the consolidated NTPR program began cleaning up the participant files. That means that the initial participant data should have been nearly complete and free of the classification errors experienced with the earlier study.

Nevertheless, we have taken additional steps to assure the quality of the participant identification process. This process included a comparison between the current (1994) data set and the 1986 data set, as well as comparisons with two other sources of participation information—a roster of CROSSROADS participants from the National Association of Atomic Veterans (NAAV) and a roster compiled from direct solicitation of information from veterans by MFUA.

METHODOLOGY

Comparison to Previous Versions of the Participant Roster

By comparing the current participant data set to the 1986 version and seeking verification of participation for sampled individuals, we were able to estimate a crude false positive rate and better understand changes that have occurred in the participant cohort over time. We drew a sample of 50 participants from each of the following categories:

- Participants who were found in both the 1986 participant list and in the current, 1994, participant list (*matched,* n = 39,844). Matched participants were defined by a corresponding first and last name and other confirmatory information such as military service number, date of birth, and unit of assignment. Allowances were made for obvious typographical errors (for example, "Johsnson, John" was accepted as a match to "Johnson, John" if there was also a match on service number or other confirming evidence).
- Participants who are currently in the study but could not be matched to a 1986 participant (n = 2,713; *new-only's*).
- Participants who were in the study in 1986 but could not be matched to a participant in the 1994 file (n = 667; *old-only's*).

MFUA requested documentation from NTPR to verify the status of each of the selected individuals. We then categorized every putative participant as a verified participant, a verified nonparticipant, or a person whose participation could not be verified using written documentary sources. To get a false positive rate we then calculated the fraction of inappropriately classified participants in the *matched* and *new-only* samples.

Comparison of Participant Roster to National Association of Atomic Veterans (NAAV) Mortality Study List

Estimating the number of persons erroneously left out of the study was more difficult than verifying the participation of those whose names were already known to be on the participant list. To estimate the false negative rate—

that is, the proportion of actual CROSSROADS participants who have been incorrectly excluded from the study—we needed to find participants who were unknown. We used two sources to find these additional participants.

NAAV provided us with a list of veterans (n = 1,251) who reported service in Operation CROSSROADS. Using this list as a benchmark, we estimated a false negative rate by matching the NAAV participants against those in our current data set, using the criteria presented above. NAAV participants were classified as either "matches" or "insufficient data."

The NAAV database was compiled by Mr. Boley Caldwell, director, NAAV Medical History Survey, from a number of medical surveys NAAV conducted on its members. The latest questionnaire was circulated in 1992 and is included in Appendix A along with Mr. Caldwell's comments on the data collection methods. Because there was insufficient time to obtain approval for follow-up, we have not attempted to contact individual veterans to verify or obtain additional identifying information. We have accepted the NAAV database as it was presented to us, editing only as necessary to ensure consistency of format in fields such as data of birth and to eliminate obvious duplicate records.

The NAAV benchmark represents a highly selective population, since it is based upon health surveys that were intended to determine potentially radiogenic mortality and morbidity among the atomic veterans. It is conceivable that veterans in the database may have been more likely to have contacted the NTPR program or the VA and, consequently, are more likely to be on our list of participants. To avoid this possible bias, we also sought participants through sources that were not connected with NAAV.

Comparison of DNA Participant Roster to a List of Participants Solicited through Veterans' Journals

In order to obtain a group of veterans for comparison who were not associated with NAAV, we placed announcements of the CROSSROADS study in several veterans' publications.[28] We included the *NAAV Newsletter* for completeness and to see if NAAV responses would be different from the others. The publications that published our announcement (in some form) included:

- *Journal of the Veterans of Foreign Wars,*
- *Journal of the American Legion,*
- *Journal of the Retired Enlisted Association,* and
- *The NAAV Newsletter.*

---

[28]We also asked for responses from veterans who participated in any of the "Five Series" of nuclear tests for the revision of the 1985 NRC study mentioned above.

With the exception of the *NAAV Newsletter*, we were limited to a few lines of text inviting a response from CROSSROADS veterans. The magazines edited the announcement to suit their needs for format and availability of space. The NAAV accommodated us with a half-page form for their readers to fill out and send in. That enabled us to distinguish between respondents who were newsletter recipients, and most likely members of NAAV, and those who were not.

We asked veterans of CROSSROADS to provide us with personal identification information and details of their participation. We refer to this as the *write-in* verification sample. This group (n = 477) was treated like the NAAV sample, but hopefully constitutes a less selective (and potentially less biased) comparison group. Because more data were available for individuals in the *write-in* group, we were able to classify them in more detail when we matched them to the 1994 participant file:

- "Matches" corresponded to individuals in the NTPR participant file as defined above.
- "Probable participants" included those who provided sufficient documentation (orders, "participation cards," narrative that indicated participation in the test, etc.).
- "Not-CROSSROADS" included individuals who mentioned the CROSSROADS study in their correspondence, but provided documentation of participation that definitely placed them at a different time and place—most often in another atomic test in the Pacific such as CASTLE (1954).
- "Unknown," which included:

—"Possible post-CROSSROADS." These individuals indicated participation during dates that were outside the operational period of CROSSROADS, but they may have been included as participants in the posttest period. Posttest participants are not included in this study as noted in Chapter 6.

—"Possible Kwajalein/Enewetak." These individuals told us of their assignment on Kwajalein or Enewetak Atolls during the operational period of CROSSROADS. Kwajalein was about 300 miles southeast of ground zero for the test and was both a staging area for test personnel and a garrison for military personnel not connected with CROSSROADS. Participation for military personnel assigned to Kwajalein depended upon whether they were assigned to a CROSSROADS unit or to a nonparticipating garrison unit. Enewetak is about 200 miles west of ground zero; the same participation rules apply.

—"Insufficient information." These individuals did not provide enough information to classify them into one of the above categories. Typically, these responders provided only last name and initials or a nickname, with no other identifying information.

Individual Follow-Up on Putative Participants of Uncertain Status

As a final quality assurance measure, we sought additional participation information on the NAAV (n = 90)[29] and *write-in* (n = 17) individuals whom we could not positively identify as either participants or nonparticipants. We sent identifying information for these 107 individuals to DNA, and asked for verification of participant status through a search of the NTPR database and personnel records.

RESULTS

Comparison with an Earlier Version of the Participant Roster

Participants Found in Both 1986 and Current Data Sets

Among the 50 individuals sampled from participants that were in both the 1986 and current data sets, 49 were found to be in the study. One was found to be an error; he had been transferred to a non-CROSSROADS unit on 30 June 1946, the day before the first detonation.

Participants Found Only in the Current Data Set—New-Only's

Among the sample of 50 *new-only* participants whose names were found in the present study, but could not be found in the 1986 data, 45 were confirmed as new participants. For one, documentation found during the validation process indicated that the individual left active duty with the Navy in November 1945 and would not have been at CROSSROADS. For another participant, the record search revealed no data that could absolutely confirm or deny participation. Three (3) individuals were not assigned duties in the CROSSROADS test but were passengers in transit aboard the PANAMINT, a CROSSROADS-participating ship. These "in transit" personnel will be discussed later in detail.

In summary, the review of the newly added participants resulted in 48 being confirmed (includes the 3 PANAMINT passengers), 1 erroneously included, and 1 unverifiable.

---

[29]One of these 90 discrepancies was a duplicate record, which left 89 unique records for analysis.

Participants Found Only in the 1986 Data Set—Old-Only's

Of the sample of 50 participants found only in the 1986 list, and not matched to the current participant list, 26 (52 percent) were still participants. They had not matched until their identification information (spelling of name or service number) had been corrected during clean-up. Another comparably sized group of 23 (46 percent) were confirmed deletions for the following reasons:

- one was an "in transit" case, as described above.
- thirteen were deleted during the clean-up of the CROSSROADS data when information indicated they were elsewhere during the test.
- nine were deleted during clean-up when their units were found not to have met eligibility criteria.

The remaining individual was identified only by last name and initials of first and middle name. Although he appears on both old and new CROSSROADS rosters as a participant, the lack of definitive identification prevents absolute confirmation of his status.

NTPR estimated that there should have been only 100 participants eliminated from the study between 1986 and 1994. Hence, NTPR was justifiably concerned that we found 667 individuals in the old data set who could not be matched, with certainty, to the current one. They also agreed to investigate the validity of the remaining 617, in addition to providing documentation on the 50 sampled *old-only's*. The final status of the remaining 617 are shown in Table E-1.

TABLE E-1. Resolution of 617 Apparent Participant Deletions Between 1986 and 1994

No. of Apparent Deletions	%	Resolution of Participant Status
333	54	In the participant list with corrected identification data
273	44	Validated deletions—new data contradicted participation
7	1	Erroneous deletions
4	1	Records not available at time of writing or insufficient information available for positive identification
617	100	Total personnel researched

Of the seven erroneous deletions, three were Marines who were assigned to CROSSROADS but stationed on Kwajalein Atoll (see discussion above of “Possible Kwajalein/Enewetak” participant). Three were found to have been assigned to participating Navy ships. One was noted as a validated deletion without further annotation.

Comparison with the NAAV Medical Survey

Of the 1,251 veterans in the NAAV Medical Survey who indicated participation in CROSSROADS, we were able to match all but 89 to our current participant list. For these 89 individuals we had insufficient information to declare them a match.

Comparison with the Write-in List

The amount of information provided by those who responded to our publication inquiry varied widely. Some veterans provided detailed documentation of their participation, including both official government documents and their own narrative description of events they witnessed. Others provided only their name and a statement that they were present at CROSSROADS.

In all, we received 477 responses that mentioned CROSSROADS in one way or another. When we matched the respondents to our participant list, we obtained the results shown in Table E-2. Respondents who used the NAAV form are tabulated separately from those who responded by letter or other written means.

TABLE E-2. Summary of Completeness of the NTPR Participant List as Indicated by Veteran Responses to MFUA Solicitations Published in Veterans' Publications

Match Status	NAAV* Form Respondents	Other Respondents	Total No. of Respondents
Matched to Participant File	174	271	445
Not in CROSSROADS	5	10	15
Probable Participant, not listed on the file	0	7	7
Unknown—Possible Enewetak Participant	1	0	1
Unknown—Possible Kwajalein Participant	0	3	3
Unknown—Possible Post Participant	1	2	3
Unknown—Insufficient Information	0	3	3
Total Number of Respondents	181	296	477

*Those respondents who replied by means of a form published by the NAAV in their newsletter.

Follow-Up on Putative Participants of Uncertain Status

Of the 107 individuals we sent to DNA for individual verification of status, 1 was found to be a duplicate and 3 were found on both the NAAV and *write-in* lists. Of the 103 unique records, DNA provided participation information summarized in Table E-3.

TABLE E-3. Disposition of 103 Records of Putative Participants in CROSSROADS Whose Status was Uncertain

No. of Individuals	Disposition
1	Newly identified navy participant who went to the CROSSROADS operational area but was not on the muster roll of the ship to which he was assigned. Participation was ascertained by reference to individual's personnel record.
1	Newly identified Army Air Corps participant assigned to Kwajalein. Not assigned to operation CROSSROADS *per se*, but his personnel jacket noted he flew missions in support of the operation. He therefore qualifies as a participant.
1	Newly identified Navy participant assigned to Naval Air Station, Kwajalein. He had administrative duties on Kwajalein in support of CROSSROADS and therefore qualifies as a participant.
1	New Navy participant whose service record shows he was assigned to Naval Air Base Kwajalein in support of CROSSROADS.
65	Non-participants who had personnel records showing duties with non-CROSSROADS units during the operational period. Many of these were identified as participants in other nuclear tests, most frequently SANDSTONE (1948).
19	Unknown. Personnel records were not available, because they were burned or there was insufficient information available to retrieve a record.
15	Confirmed as participants and found on the MFUA study roster based on name match. These individuals are considered by DNA to be participants, and are in the MFUA study file. They were not initially matched because of unrecognized typographical errors in the source list (ex. Vonname should have been Von Name).
103	Total records considered

The final disposition of the 89 discrepancies from the NAAV Medical Survey list are summarized in Table E-4.

TABLE E-4. Disposition of 89 Discrepant Records from the NAAV Medical Survey List

Disposition	Count
Matched to participant file	10
Newly identified CROSSROADS participants	3
Civilians in CROSSROADS but not in the study	2
Post-CROSSROADS participant	1
On MFUA study roster but found ineligible	1
Not in CROSSROADS[a]	57
Unknown[b]	15
Total	89

[a]These individuals were assigned duties elsewhere during the CROSSROADS operational period. Several were found at tests other than CROSSROADS; SANDSTONE, 1948, was common.
[b]Personnel records could not be found for these individuals to verify or disallow participation.

With the additional data provided by DNA on the 17 unresolved cases in Table E-2, we were able to collapse the *write-in* data as shown in Table E-5.

TABLE E-5. Summary of Completeness of the NTPR Participant List According to *Write-in* Data (includes verification of 17 discrepancies by personnel record searches at DNA)

Match Status	NAAV Respondents	*Write-in* Respondents	Total No. of Respondents
Matched to participant roster	174	272	446
Newly identified participant	0	1	1
Not in CROSSROADS[a]	6	20	26
Unknown[b]	1	3	4
Total number of respondents	181	296	477

[a]These individuals were assigned duties elsewhere during the CROSSROADS operational period. Several were found at tests other than CROSSROADS; SANDSTONE, 1948, was common.
[b]Personnel records could not be found for these individuals to verify or disallow participation.

DISCUSSION

The vast majority (93.6 percent) of participants in the old CROSSROADS data set (1986) matched with the new (1994). Based upon our evaluation of the validation data, the primary reasons for mismatches were clean-up of identification information (service number, name spelling, etc.) and deletion of individuals (or units) whose participation was contradicted by new information. To determine the approximate numbers of participants who have been deleted and added to the study since 1986, we needed to correct for the participants who were currently in both the *old-only* and *new-only* categories because of corrections in identification information that prevented their matching. Using estimated proportions of verified and deleted participants, available in Table E-2, we estimated the actual numbers of participants added to and deleted from the study to be approximately 2,250 (5.3 percent) and 375 (0.9 percent) respectively. The remaining 0.2 percent is accounted for by erroneous deletions and by individuals for whom insufficient information exists to make a definitive determination of participant status.

Among the sample of 50 *matched* and 50 *new-only* participants, one individual in each group was found to be erroneously classified as a participant. One *new-only* had no records available and was classified as *unknown*. Based on the combined data for *matched* and *new-only* data, we estimate the false inclusion rate to be 2 percent or 3 percent, depending upon the status of the *unknown* participant.

We have included as confirmed participants, three *new-only* individuals who were "in transit" aboard the PANAMINT (AGC-13). These warrant special attention since they illustrate a point about the inclusion criteria for participation in CROSSROADS. Inclusion in the CROSSROADS participant list is primarily an administrative decision intended for compensation purposes and is not based on documented exposure to radiation (see note 10). The "in transit" individuals were not assigned duties in the CROSSROADS test, but were given passage aboard a CROSSROADS-participating ship.

The VA addresses the question of passengers as follows (VA 1993):

> Persons whose only potential for exposure arose from passage on *contaminated* vessels would be deemed to have 'onsite participation' . . . if they were passengers during an official operational period [emphasis added].

Initially, lacking a definition of "contaminated," NTPR considered these PANAMINT passengers to be participants. This appears reasonable, because the ship did not receive its official radiological clearance until 22 November 1946, well after the operational period of the test. However, the PANAMINT had an assigned dose of 0.00 Sv (0.00 rem) (i.e., those aboard received no radiation dose as a result of their presence on the ship). In July 1995, based on this dose, NTPR determined that PANAMINT did not appear to satisfy the "contaminated" ship criteria. Therefore, its passengers were designated nonparticipants. For our purposes, we have left these (approximately 50)[30] "in transit" personnel in the study, maintaining their classification as participants as of the freeze date of our data set (28 February 1995).[31]

We derived the missing participant rate (false negatives) by comparing the NTPR participant list to individuals on the *write-in* list compiled from publication advertisements and to those on the NAAV Medical Survey list. Because many of the *write-in* veterans provided detailed data in response to our solicitation, the process of matching them to the participant roster may have been somewhat more reliable than it was for the NAAV Medical Survey. As a result of this, and perhaps other factors, the fraction of exact matches was slightly higher for the *write-in* analysis—93.3 percent for the *write-in* vs. 92.8 percent for the NAAV Medical Survey.

Several individuals in the *write-in* sample (n = 477) provided evidence that they were actually **not** in CROSSROADS. Removing those respondents, we were left with a denominator of 462 potential participants. If we assume the worst, that all of the *unknown* and *probable* cases were true participants, then our false negative rate is 3.7 percent (17/462). On the other hand, if we assume the best case, that only the *probable* cases (n = 7) were actually left out, and that the other *unknowns* (n = 10) are not participants, we have a false negative rate of 1.5 percent (7/452). Thus, based on this data, the actual completeness of the 1994 participant file probably lies between 96 and 98 percent.

Of the total *write-in* responses we received, 38 percent were on forms from the *NAAV Newsletter*, while the remaining 62 percent were letters. Interestingly, **none** of those who may have been inadvertently left out of the study (*probable* participants, n = 7) were NAAV respondents. It is also interesting that the completeness as indicated by the NAAV responses is higher (99.4 percent) than completeness indicated by the non-NAAV responses (94.8 percent).

In evaluating the inclusion and exclusion figures cited above, it is important to consider the assumptions we have made in deriving them. Where there was doubt, we have erred to the side that would maximize the appearance of error in the completeness of the data set.

Unless otherwise stated, if an individual's participation could not be verified, his inclusion was considered an error.

If an individual did not match with name and other confirmatory information, he was considered a nonmatch. There are individuals in this category that have first and last name matches to the current participant list, but

---

[30]Personal communication with D. M. Schaeffer. Director, NTPR, 14 March 1996.

[31]The NTPR database is constantly being updated as new participants are found and additional data on current participants are added. To maintain the integrity of the study during mortality follow-up and analysis, we did not accept any changes to the participant roster after the "freeze" date.

who have no other confirming data. These could be valid matches, but are not counted as such.

We have assumed that all the information we have been given by the veterans and the NAAV are completely accurate. In fact, there may be misspellings of names or errors in transcription of identification numbers that prevented individuals from matching our participant list.

In summary, there are two important points to be made. First, the use of participants from the 1994 file is thoroughly justified. Overwhelming proportions of both matched (to the 1986 file) and *new-only* participants in the random-sample verification were shown by documentary evidence to have been at CROSSROADS. A significant proportion of *old-only* subjects were confirmed nonparticipants, and most of the remainder were actually found in the 1994 file, only with modified (presumably corrected) identifying information.

Second, a check of the completeness of the CROSSROADS file using information independent of the administrative systems that provided our participant data showed a high level of completeness of the participant roster. Around 93–99 percent of subjects who made independent claims of participation in CROSSROADS were found on the study roster. The proportion is even higher for the respondents to the advertisement if one excludes the few confused cases in which the subjects were probably in the area at the time of the tests but do not fit the precise administrative criteria for official CROSSROADS participation (see Chapter 6).

Above, we established the completeness of the study roster independent of the DNA-NTPR program. If we now consider the new information provided by DNA on the 103 unresolved discrepancies (Table E-3), our estimates of missing participants change somewhat. The estimate from the NAAV Medical Survey list (counting *all* nonmatches as missing participants) suggested a 7 percent missing participant rate. From the more detailed data available in Table E-4, we can count 10 individuals as being matched to study participants; 61, non-CROSSROADS; and 18, missed participants (3 newly identified plus 15 still unknown). That yields, based on the NAAV Medical Survey List, a missing participant rate of 1.5 percent (18/[1251-61]).

The *write-in* data yield similar results when adjusted for the additional follow-up information in Table E-5. DNA-NTPR found one new (i.e., missing) participant and was unable to find any records on four others. Twenty-six were described as not in CROSSROADS. Based upon those data, the missing participant rate becomes 1.1 percent (5/[477-26]).

In these revised calculations, we have removed the non-CROSSROADS individuals (10, NAAV; 26, *write-ins*) from consideration. We do that with some caution. Although it is unlikely, information that could have indicated a temporary assignment to CROSSROADS may not have been entered in, or may be missing from, personnel records. If some of these individuals had undocumented CROSSROADS participation, our estimates of completeness will be toward the low end of the range cited above. But, we have retained *all* of the remaining unknown cases as missing participants, which tends to inflate the missing rate. In summary, the additional follow-up by DNA-NTPR suggests that the participant capture rate may be toward the high end of the 93–99 percent range.

CONCLUSION

We estimate that fewer than 2–4 percent of the current participants included in the NTPR data set may not actually be CROSSROADS participants (i.e., they are false positives). We are also confident that the data captures between 93 and 99 percent of those who were actually CROSSROADS participants. Since we were conservative in matching purported participants to the NTPR participant list, erring on the side of exclusion, the inclusion rate could actually be higher. If additional follow-up information provided by DNA-NTPR is considered, the capture rate would be toward the upper end of the range. In short, there is no evidence from any of the above sources that the roster of CROSSROADS participants studied by MFUA is deficient in a substantial manner.

F

Verification of Completeness and Accuracy of Mortality Ascertainment

ASSESSMENT OF COMPLETENESS

We describe the procedural steps, along with success rates, involved (Table F-1) in determining vital status information about the 73,910 Navy personnel considered in most of this study's analyses.

The comparison of missing rates for the participants and controls informs about the possible *influence* these gaps might have on the statistics calculated and inferences drawn from them.

TABLE F-1. Procedural Steps and Success Rates for Determination of Vital Status Information

Procedural Step	Participants (38,668), %	Controls (35,242), %	Total No.	Total %
All submitted to BIRLS	100.0	100.0	73,910	100.0
Of those submitted to BIRLS, % found on BIRLS	87.4	88.1		87.7
Of those found on BIRLS, % with indication of death	38.7	37.9		38.3
Of those with indication on BIRLS of death, indicated by				
% date of death	96.9	96.9		96.9
% FARC folder location only	3.1	3.1		3.1
Of those with indication on BIRLS of death, % with claims folder location noted in BIRLS	80.3	81.3		80.8
Of those with claims folder location noted on BIRLS,				
% in VA regional offices	71.1	70.7		70.9
% in FARCs	28.6	29.3		28.9
Submitted to VAMI	100.0	100.0	24,762	100.0
Of those submitted to VAMI, % found	92.6	91.3		91.9

A veteran could be "not found" on the Beneficiary Identification and Locator Subsystem (BIRLS) for varied reasons: (a) the record existed but the Medical Follow-up Agency (MFUA) submitted insufficient information, such as a misspelled name, to identify it; (b) the requesting information was correct but the BIRLS record includes a misspelling; (c) a veteran was not entered into BIRLS because the veteran or a surviving dependent had filed no claim for medical, educational, loan, death, or other benefits. Similarly, a claims folder—identified by BIRLS—could be "not found" because (a) the request went to the wrong VA Regional Office (VARO), (b) misfiling, (c) the file was transferred to another VARO, or (d) the file was transferred to a regional Archives center (FARC). Finally, a claims folder may be found yet not contain the death certificate, the cause of death, or have been unusable because of an illegible or poorly copied certificate.

Completeness of Mortality Follow-Up

The completeness of follow-up is displayed in Tables F-2 and F-3 below.

TABLE F-2. Vital Status for Navy Personnel

Vital Status	Participants		Controls		All	
	No.	%	No.	%	No.	%
Dead	12,092	31.3	10,804	30.8	22,896	31.1
Alive	21,771	56.3	20,321	58.0	42,092	57.1
LTFU	4,805	12.4	3,911	11.2	8,716	11.8
Total	38,668	100.0	35,036	100.0	73,704	100.0

TABLE F-3. Completeness of Mortality Information

Vital Status Information	Participants		Controls		All	
	No.	%	No.	%	No.	%
Cause and Date	10,436	86.3	9,649	89.3	20,085	87.7
Cause only	7	0.1	10	0.1	17	0.1
Date only	1,639	13.6	1,135	10.5	2,774	12.1
Neither	10	0.1	10	0.1	20	0.1
Total dead	12,092	100	10,804	100	22,896	100

ASSESSMENT OF VALIDITY

Mortality Ascertainment

To assess the quality of VA records' vital status information, we did an independent search of two federal, non-VA, databases. While none of the three is designated as the correct standard, similar findings would support the validity of each of them.

HCFA

All Lost-to-follow-up (LTFU) and a sample of Alive and Dead participants and controls were searched in Health Care Financing Administration (HCFA) files (Table F-4). Since HCFA does not record deaths prior to Medicare eligibility, we expected to find an undercount of deaths in "Dead" and an overcount in "LTFU." Deaths before 1976 are extremely unlikely to be picked up, as are deaths before age 65. Because HCFA is concerned with medical benefits to living enrollees, its data are unlikely to confirm as "Alive" someone who is dead.

TABLE F-4. Summary of Vital Status for Study Records Submitted to HCFA

Vital Status from VA/MFUA Records	Participants	Controls	All
Alive	1,035	891	1,926
Dead	1,060	964	2,024
Lost to follow-up	5,649	6,160	11,809
Total	7,744	8,015	15,759

Methods. The HCFA enrollment files used in this examination of VA mortality ascertainment are of two kinds. The first kind of file is a called an "alpha search file" and the second a "vital status file." Both files contain information about HCFA beneficiaries, primarily Medicare beneficiaries, and their vital status. Other than formatting, the practical difference between the files is that the first is searched using a subject's name and date of birth, while the second uses the Social Security Number (SSN).

For this examination of the completeness of VA mortality reporting, all participants and controls who were lost to VA follow-up (i.e., LTFU, no record in the BIRLS file) as of July 1995 were matched against HCFA enrollment files, as were random samples of about 1,000 presumed dead and presumed alive from both participants and controls. All subjects in this exercise were matched against the alpha search file, and subjects with SSN were also matched against the vital status file.

The central, practical methodological issue is the definition of a match. Because there were multiple matches against the alpha search and vital status files, a scheme was developed to identify and classify the "best" match for any single subject. Because everyone was matched against the alpha search file, matches against it were considered first, and only if there was no "good" (see below) match against the alpha search file were matches against the vital status file considered. HCFA's algorithm for matching the alpha search file looks at the matches between various data elements and assigns point scores for each individual matching element. The data elements matched and their respective point scores are as follows: last name (64 points), month of birth (32 points), sex (16 points), first name (8 points), year of birth (4 points), day of birth (2 points), and middle initial (1 point). Sex was not included on our input file, so HCFA awarded no points for matching that element on any individual.

Matching scores ranged from a maximum of 111 points (all elements matched, save sex) to zero (no elements matched). Practically speaking, however, matching scores sorted themselves into two obvious groups: 104 points or more (i.e., from last name, first name, and month of birth matches up through perfect matches) and 103 points or less. Roughly three-quarters of the 23,200 potential matching records file fell into the first category, with the other one-quarter in the second group. Thus, we considered a good match to be a match associated with a point score of 104 or more. In addition, because we provided an SSN on the alpha search file whenever available, it was possible to check the SSN we provided with the SSN returned by HCFA. When these SSNs were different, the match was discarded as "bad," no matter what the matching score was.

After being matched against the alpha search file process, many subjects still remained unmatched. If a subject had no match or a bad match, the vital status (SSN search) file was consulted. If there was an exact match between SSN and last name on the vital status file, that record was considered a good match and added to the file. The results tabulated below are based on the results of the combined alpha search and vital status file matching.

Results. Table F-5 shows the results of the HCFA file matching process. Each of the three groups defined on the basis of VA follow-up (Lost-to-Follow-Up, Alive, and Dead) is shown separately for participants and controls. In this table, deaths after the study mortality cut-off date (31 December 1992) were counted as "Dead." Subsequent tables in this chapter limit "Dead" to veterans who died within the study period.

The LTFU constitute the largest groups of participants and controls. Roughly 80 percent of participant LTFU and 70 percent of control LTFU were matched at HCFA. Disregarding nonmatches, the overwhelming proportion of LTFU were found alive on HCFA: 84.7 percent for participants and 82.7 percent for controls (see discussion below).

Roughly 85 percent of living participants and controls in the random sample were matched at HCFA. Again disregarding nonmatches, the overwhelming proportion of these subjects were found alive on HCFA: 92.1 percent for participants and 95.3 percent for controls. Results for the random sample of VA deaths were much different than for the other groups. Only about 55 percent of Dead participants in the random sample were found at HCFA, compared to around 40 percent of controls. Again disregarding nonmatches, there is still a general validation of the VA data: two-thirds of the participants were found dead on HCFA and three-quarters of controls. Possible reasons for the high number of nonmatches among deaths are discussed below.

Discussion. In general, vital status data from HCFA validated the VA results. Disregarding nonmatches, the overwhelming proportion of subjects shown dead by the VA were dead according to HCFA; the same was true for living subjects. In addition, the LTFU group has now been shown to consist mostly of living individuals (about 8 percent were dead).

TABLE F-5. Comparison of VA and HCFA Vital Status for Operation CROSSROADS Participants and Controls

MFUA Status	HCFA Status	Participants Number	Participants % of Total	Participants % of Matches	Controls Number	Controls % of Total	Controls % of Matches
LTFU							
	Alive	3,883	68.7%	84.7%	3628	59.0%	82.7%
	Dead*	701	12.4%	15.3%	757	12.3%	17.3%
	No match	1,065	18.9%	—	1775	28.8%	—
	TOTAL	5,649	100%	100%	6160	100%	100%
ALIVE							
	Alive	**813**	**78.6%**	**92.1%**	**731**	**82.0%**	95.3%
	Dead*	70	6.8%	7.9%	36	4.0%	4.7%
	No match	152	14.7%	—	124	13.9%	—
	TOTAL	1,035	100%	100%	891	100%	100%
DEAD							
	Alive	143	13.5%	24.9%	39	4.0%	10.8%
	Dead*	**431**	**40.7%**	**75.1%**	**323**	**33.5%**	89.2%
	No match	486	45.8%	—	602	62.4%	—
	TOTAL	1,060	100%	100%	964	100%	100%

*In this table, deaths after the study mortality cut-off date (12/31/92) counted as "Dead." Subsequent tables in this appendix limit "Dead" to veterans who died within the study period.

Two additional topics merit some further discussion. First, deaths occurring early in the follow-up may have occurred before the decedent could have been enrolled as a HCFA beneficiary (for example, at age 65, for Medicare), and so *should not* have been found in the HCFA files. This seems the most likely explanation for the low finding among decedents.

Lastly, the fact that the bulk of LTFU were found alive on HCFA could have been predicted. A number of studies (Beebe and Simon 1969, Page 1992, Page et al. 1995) have shown that VA death reporting is roughly 95 percent complete for World War II veterans. Add to this an estimated death rate of around 30 percent and a LTFU rate of 15 percent, and the arithmetic works out as follows. In a group of some 1,000 World War II veterans, 700 will be living and 300 dead. Of the 300 dead, 285 (95 percent) are known to BIRLS and 15 (5 percent) unknown. Of the one thousand, 850 (85 percent) will be found on BIRLS and 150 (15 percent) LTFU. From this, it can be determined that there are only 15 LTFU deaths among the total of 150 LTFU subjects, a rate of 10 percent, which is one-third of the overall death rate and consistent with our HCFA data. That the bulk of LTFU in our sample were confirmed alive is thus as one would have expected.

NDI

With related but different accuracy checks in mind, we submitted all 4,107 deaths for which, at the time, we had no death certificate (and, therefore, no cause of death) and which occurred after the National Death Index (NDI) had started (1979) and before the study follow-up cut-off date (31 December 1992). These were sent to obtain information needed to get death certificates from state vital statistics offices. We also sent a sample (about 250 in each category) of alive and dead participants and controls for verification of death status.

Our NDI request, unlike the limitations in our expectations of HCFA data, was therefore structured so that all MFUA-classified "Dead" records should be found as "Dead" on NDI. However, we would expect some of the MFUA-classified "Alive" and a larger portion of the MFUA-classified "LTFU" to be in the NDI database as "Dead." The reason is that for the former we had some positive information in BIRLS indicating a death had not occurred, while for the latter we had no information.

NDI characterized the 5,108 records MFUA submitted as involved in matches, nonmatching, and rejected. Of those matching, user (MFUA) records could match to one or more NDI records (see distribution in Table F-6).

TABLE F-6. Number of Potential Matches for Each Record Submitted to NDI

No. of NDI Matches Returned for Each Record Submitted	No. of MFUA Records Submitted
1 NDI record	2,259
2 NDI records	646
3	386
4	230
5	150
6	109
7	90
8	71
9	53
10	41
≥11 NDI records	424
MFUA records involved in matches	4,459
Nonmatching user records	540
Records rejected	9
Total submitted by user	5,108

Of 5,108 records MFUA sent, NDI proposed at least one match for 4,459. MFUA accepted 3,656 as "good" for this analysis. The remaining 803 MFUA records with at least one NDI match can be—but have not been—reviewed by hand/eye to judge discrepancies. The results of the NDI search are shown in Table F-7. There were also 803 "questionable matches,"some of which would probably be found to be correct, that is, "Dead," on NDI. The percentages in columns 4, 7, and 10 would then go up; view them as lower bounds.

EXTERNAL VALIDATION DISCUSSION

Mortality Information

Despite our sending different samples, different years of coverage, and different technical approaches to matching, NDI and HCFA results are consistent with each other for both those we considered alive and those who were Lost-to-Follow-Up (Table F-8).

Of participants for whom MFUA records would indicate vital status as "Alive," HCFA and NDI each found 3.6 percent to be "Dead" (positive information in their databases indicating a death). Both data sources reported fewer controls in this category (NDI, 1.2 percent; HCFA, 2.2 percent).

TABLE F-7. Comparison of NDI and MFUA Mortality Information

	Participants			Controls			Total		
		On NDI (= dead)			On NDI (= dead)			On NDI (= dead)	
MFUA Status	Submitted	No.	%*	Submitted	No.	%	Submitted	No.	%
Alive	251	9	3.6	250	3	1.2	501	12	2.4
Dead	2,430	2,112	86.9	1,677	1,491	88.9	4,107	3,603	87.7
LTFU	250	22	8.8	250	19	7.6	500	41	8.2
Total	2,931	2,143		2,177	1,513		5,108	3,656	

*Of the 803 "questionable matches," some would probably be found to be correct, that is, "Dead," on NDI. The percentages in columns 4, 7, and 10 would then go up; view them as lower bounds.

TABLE F-8. NDI and HCFA Comparisons

MFUA Status →	Participants		Controls	
External Response	NDI	HCFA	NDI	HCFA
Alive → Dead	3.6%	3.6%	1.2%	2.2%
Dead → Dead	86.9%	34.2%	88.9%	28.3%
LTFU → Dead	8.8%	7.3%	7.6%	7.8%

HCFA was created in the 1970s to oversee the financial management of the Medicaid and, later, the Medicare programs. Its quality is maintained for current administrative purposes, and data are updated if the information might be relevant to benefits decisions; hence, recent deaths are well recorded (tied with the stopping of Social Security benefits), but earlier ones might not be. While the HCFA data were consistent with expectations and therefore somewhat informative, they are not a good fit for a mortality study covering substantial deaths before 1980 such as the CROSSROADS study. Less than a third of MFUA-considered "Dead" were reported as "Dead" based on the HCFA enrollment tapes; many deaths occurred in our study cohort before 1980.

Vital status records at two databases external to VA confirm our expectation that individuals we label "Lost to follow-up" are probably "Alive." Looking at controls and participants together, NDI reported as "Dead" 2.4 percent of individuals MFUA considered Alive, 8.2 percent of these MFUA considered LTFU, and 87.7 percent of those MFUA considered "Dead." For those categories, HCFA reported a similar trend with lower values (see preceding paragraph). Therefore, we believe we are not introducing large additional bias into our analyses by considering the LTFU individuals to be "not dead."

Cause-of-Death Information

To evaluate the reliability of cause-of-death coding according to the ICD-9 classification system, we submitted already coded death certificates to a contract nosologist for recoding without identifying them as other than routine (Table F-9). Because of specific concerns about the coding of leukemia, an endpoint of radiation exposure, all 166 death certificates available at the time noting leukemia were recoded, along with all records noting hematopoietic or lymphatic cancers. All records noting other diseases of the blood and blood-forming organs were also included to check whether any leukemias may have been so coded. Also recoded was a sample of death certificates indicating all other malignant neoplasms, noncancer disease deaths, and external causes of deaths.

TABLE F-9. Distribution of Causes of Death for 641 Death Certificates Sent for Recoding

No. of Death Certificates	Disease Category
166	All leukemias
244	All other hematopoietic or lymphatic cancers
30	All other diseases of the blood and blood-forming organs
102	Sample of all other malignant neoplasms
83	Sample of noncancer disease deaths
16	Sample of external causes of death

Of the 410 records sent for recoding because they were initially coded as leukemia (ICD9 204.0–208.9) or other lymphopoietic cancer (ICD9 200.0–203.8)[32] as the underlying cause of death, there were 33 discrepant pairs. Nineteen of those discrepancies did not affect the cause-of-death analysis category to which we would have assigned the case in our analyses. The remaining 14 discrepancies fit into 3 groups:

- Five (5) discrepancies involved moving from one lymphopoietic cancer category to another (e.g., leukemia to cancer of other lymphatic tissue)—so analysis of the combined lymphopoietic cancer group would not have been affected, although each specific category would have been.
- Four (4) discrepancies involved moving from a lymphopoietic cancer category to another disease category that we will explore in the study analyses (e.g., multiple myeloma to disease of the circulatory system)—so the deaths would be considered in the analysis, but not as lymphopoietic cancer deaths.
- Five (5) discrepancies involved moving from a lymphopoietic cancer category to a disease category that will not be separately considered in this study (e.g., cancer of other lymphatic tissue to herpes zoster)—so the deaths would be included only in the "all-cause" category.

Considering leukemias alone, there were 18 discrepant pairs (18/166 = 10.4 percent). Only one of these affected the analysis category (leukemia and aleukemia), with that case moving from leukemia to the more general all lymphopoietic cancers. In an analysis of leukemias alone, this death (1/166 = 0.6 percent) would have been missed. Conversely, one death coded originally as lymphosarcoma or reticulosarcoma was recoded as a leukemia. The comparisons we make here between codings only identify discrepancies; they do not show which of each pair is correct.

Other proportions support a similar view of discrepancies:

[32]Code ranges chosen to match the NCI mortality tables (NCI 1995).

- Of the lymphopoietic cancer deaths, 8.0 percent (33/410) had discrepancies in the coded underlying cause of death. All others matched exactly.
- A smaller proportion—3.4 percent (14/410)—of the lymphopoietic cancer deaths had discrepancies in the coded underlying cause of death that would have changed the cause-of-death category used in the study analyses.

Of the 201 drawn as a sample from other causes of deaths (coded as all malignant neoplasms, noncancer diseases, and external causes), 8 (4.0 percent) were in discrepancy categories that had a high likelihood of changing analysis category.

Thirty deaths from other diseases of blood and blood-forming organs (ICD9 282–289) were recoded to see whether any would turn up coded as leukemias. There were five discrepant pairs, but none of them resulted in a leukemia.